CHRONIC PAIN RESET

30 Days of Activities,
Practices, and Skills to
Help You Thrive

Afton L. Hassett, PsyD

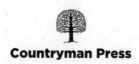

Countryman Press

An Imprint of W. W. Norton & Company
Celebrating a Century of Independent Publishing

Chronic Pain Reset was created to help you better understand the role of the brain in the experience of pain and to learn evidence-based strategies that have proven helpful for others. This book is not intended to diagnose, treat, cure, or prevent any condition or disease, or as a substitute for the medical advice of physicians.

Manufacturing by Lake Book Manufacturing
Production manager: Devon Zahn

Countryman Press
www.countrymanpress.com

An imprint of W. W. Norton & Company, Inc.
500 Fifth Avenue, New York, NY 10110
www.wwnorton.com

978-1-68268-765-9

10 9 8 7 6 5 4 3 2 1

To my parents, whom I adore.

For my mom, Linda, who thinks it's perfectly reasonable to soak dirty sneakers in a bidet, and my dad, Ramon, who always went out to "fancy dinner" with a jalapeño in his suit pocket.

*My quirks can be explained by genetics **and** environment.*

CONTENTS

Foreword by Barbara L. Fredrickson, PhD............... xi

Introduction... xv

PART ONE   YOU HAVE THE POWER TO HIT RESET.................... 1

1. Pain Is in Your Brain.. 3

2. Co-Occurring Symptoms and Conditions............... 14

3. Stress and the Price the Body Pays......................... 22

4. Thoughts Are Brain Activities.............................. 33

5. Emotions Are Physiological Events........................ 41

6. Trauma, Pain, and Healing 51

7. Mindfulness and the Power of Presence................. 60

8. Sleep, Your Fickle Friend...................................... 68

9. Exercise Is a Wonder Drug.................................... 76

10. Social Connectedness 86

11. Must Do versus Love to Do 97

12. Values, Virtues, and Strengths 106

13. Grit, Gratitude, and Grace 116

14. In Awe of Something Greater............................. 126

15. Purpose in Life and the Way Forward.................. 136

16. Preparing for Your Journey 142

PART TWO   THIRTY ACTIVITIES, PRACTICES, AND SKILLS

FOR A BETTER LIFE.. 151

DAY 1.   Paced Breathing................................. 152

DAY 2.   Progressive Muscle Relaxation.................. 154

DAY 3.   Mindful Breathing.............................. 156

DAY 4.   Guided Imagery................................. 158

DAY 5.   Savoring.. 160

DAY 6.   Healthy Sleep Habits........................... 162

DAY 7.   Time-Based Pacing.............................. 164

DAY 8.   Pleasant Activity Scheduling................... 166

DAY 9.   Walking Program 168

DAY 10.   Take a Nature Break............................ 170

DAY 11.   Show Yourself Compassion 172

DAY 12.   Thought Approach 1:
          Reframe Negative Thoughts...................... 174

DAY 13.   Thought Approach 2:
          Unhelpful Thoughts Come and Go 176

DAY 14.   Thought Approach 3: Coping Coach 178

DAY 15.   Thought Approach 4: Somatic Tracking........... 180

DAY 16. Self-Soothe 182

DAY 17. Release Painful Emotions 184

DAY 18. Embrace Positive Emotions 186

DAY 19. Music Is Emotional Medicine 188

DAY 20. Create a Relationship Tree 190

DAY 21. Daily Connection 192

DAY 22. Forgive 194

DAY 23. Acts of Kindness 196

DAY 24. The Gift of Giving 198

DAY 25. Practice Gratitude 200

DAY 26. Positive Service 202

DAY 27. Appreciate the Arts 204

DAY 28. Cultivate Purpose in Life 206

DAY 29. Best Possible Self 208

DAY 30. Take an "Aweliday" 210

PART THREE THE ROAD FORWARD 213

Create Your Thriving Plan 215

Live Your Thriving Plan 230

Acknowledgments 239

Notes 243

Resources 255

Index 259

FOREWORD

FOR THIRTY YEARS, I've worked in the science of positive emotions, focusing on how these fleeting, uplifted states relate to health and well-being. Across these decades, I've seen the evidence for the health benefits of positive emotions proliferate and provide plenty of reasons for enthusiasm and hope.

I first met Dr. Hassett in 2016, when I was president of the International Positive Psychology Association (IPPA). That society serves as the intellectual home to a diverse group of researchers, psychologists, and other healthcare professionals who gather every two years to discuss the latest advances in research and practice. At that time, Dr. Hassett and a handful of academic researchers were working to establish a division within IPPA consisting of kindred spirits who studied the physical effects of positive emotions, what they termed "positive health." That small but enthusiastic group laid the groundwork for a thriving community of people, including me, who are intrigued by the powerful effects that positive emotions, supportive relationships, and meaningful activities can have on physical health, including chronic pain.

Not long after our first meeting, I joined her team as a coinvestigator on a research grant application she was submitting to the National Institutes of Health (NIH). In this context, I learned about the important work underway at the Chronic Pain and Fatigue Research Center (CPFRC). Their pain research focused on explaining the complex role that the brain plays in the experience of pain, as well as how thoughts, emotions, and behavior impact the pain experience. Their truly groundbreaking research held the steadfast stance that chronic pain was *not* a mental health problem, as many others had claimed, but a biological condition in which the brain amplifies pain signals, making the pain feel much worse. They also showed that negative emotions and thoughts could amplify pain signals further.

As you might expect, Dr. Hassett's pioneering work considers important processes, such as depression and catastrophic thinking, and their role in amplifying pain. Yet her truly unique contribution is that she studies the buffering effects of positive emotions and the benefits of resilience for people with pain. She has shown that more resilient people report less pain and lead lives that are more active and rewarding, *despite* their pain. Indeed, Dr. Hassett is a global leader in this area. As a tenured associate professor in the Department of Anesthesiology and the director of pain and opioid research at the University of Michigan, she has addressed the National Academy of Medicine, one of the highest academic honors, and won numerous awards for her research, service, and leadership.

Her work with people with chronic pain, published across more than 100 scientific articles, aligns well with what my team and I in the Positive Emotions and Psychophysiology Laboratory (PEP Lab) have shown over the years. You see, positive emotions, fleeting as they are, fundamentally change the way your brain absorbs information. Positive emotions momentarily broaden your mindset, allowing you to see the big picture more readily. We also have discovered, through randomized trials, that when people learn to cultivate more positive-emotion moments in their days, they little-by-little grow more resilient and resourceful and show improved biomarkers of health. In recent work, we followed married couples for thirty years and found that those with the most shared moments of positive emotion had the best health trajectories and lived the longest.

Perhaps the greatest frustration of academic researchers is that we test and identify effective strategies and treatments in our labs, but too few of these ever reach the people who might benefit the most. Supported by the NIH, Dr. Hassett; her mentor, Dan Clauw, MD; and the remarkable team at the CPFRC are conducting two large clinical trials to help us understand more about who responds best to what treatment for chronic pain. These studies consider medication, but they more broadly study treatments that empower patients to take more ownership of their care, including physical therapy and exercise, mindfulness approaches, acupressure, and cognitive-behavioral therapies. Those trials will add to what we already know: that the most effective treatments seem to be the ones that make the most sense to patients and *that they're willing to do.* That principle lies at the center of *Chronic Pain Reset.* You will try and select the treatment strategies that make the most sense to you and that you might even be *excited* to do.

The first part of this book details the fascinating research that explains the neuroscience of pain, as well as how seemingly unrelated processes such as friendship, gratitude, pleasant activities, and happiness might influence pain processing in your brain. These scientifically sound chapters are short and written in a way that makes them understandable and even entertaining. Please don't skip them! Between some of the chapters, you'll find little treasures, stories written by people like you who live with chronic pain. These reflections are moving, educational, and inspirational. I hope you enjoy them as much as I do.

Then, in part two of the book, Dr. Hassett will guide you through conducting an experiment of your own. Over the course of thirty days, she will share with you one activity, practice, or skill each day and encourage you to try it. From your own firsthand experience, you'll determine the strategies that you'll make part of your life after the exploration period ends. In the last two chapters, Dr. Hassett will show you how to create a Thriving Plan to help you decrease your experience of pain and add more joy to your life for years to come.

With its impressive scope and inspiring message, this book offers a fresh perspective on pain. If you're one of the millions who live with chronic pain, count yourself fortunate to have this chance to absorb the discoveries and advice from a true expert in positive health. With practice, and with Dr. Hassett as your compassionate guide, you'll discover for yourself new ways to unlock greater ease and more spaciousness in your daily life.

Barbara L. Fredrickson, PhD

INTRODUCTION

LEFT TO ITS OWN DEVICES, chronic pain cheats, lies, and steals. It can cheat you out of the life you envisioned for yourself before it came along. It can tell you lies: you are broken, in constant danger, or worthless. It often steals from you the most important activities, goals, and people in your life, as well as your sense of independence, security, and well-being. However, because you're reading this book, you've told me that you're ready to take back your life.

As a pain psychologist, I've worked with many people with chronic pain and have learned, firsthand, about the toll it can take. Through more than two decades of research, I also have learned that many people find ways to lead productive, interesting, enjoyable lives, despite the chronic pain that they often experience every day. They have reclaimed their lives from the misleading messages of chronic pain, and you can, too.

This book consists of three equally important parts. In the first, you'll learn about the remarkable evolution of pain science over the last three decades. The data are overwhelming: pain is in the brain. Your experience of chronic pain may result partially or almost completely from changes in the structure and function of your brain. Throughout your life, your brain retains its ability to change, to rewire—a process known as neuroplasticity. Just as your brain has overlearned how to communicate pain signals, it can be taught new, more adaptive ways to function. Let's think of this strategy as initiating a brain *reset*.

In this first part of this book, a series of short chapters will help you understand how many of the seemingly unrelated activities that you will try in the second part of this book might actually work for you. Understanding how or why a pain management strategy works can make it more effective, so I've tried to make the neuroscience easy to understand. Each chapter ends with a summary of ideas to remember. What you learn in the first part of this book may help you decide which of the activities, practices, and skills could work best for you over time. Everyone has different needs and preferences. What makes complete sense to one person given their worldview and understanding of their pain will make someone else roll their eyes in disbelief. That's fine! Focus on what makes sense to *you*.

All the activities and practices in Part Two can influence or affect one part of your brain or another, building new neural connections meant to starve your pain instead of feeding it. Regardless of whether you're an enthusiastic experimenter or an eye-rolling skeptic, I ask you to be willing to embark on an adventure and consider both new and tried-and-true ideas for the thirty-day exploration period in Part Two.

Each day, you'll try something new. Every one of these offerings is based on scientific evidence, meaning that they have already been shown to be helpful for people with a variety of chronic illnesses, including chronic pain. Read and think about each activity, but more importantly, you need to *try it*. Even if you've done it or something like it before, do it again in the context of this thirty-day exploration period. At the end of each day, you'll take stock of how it went and whether you want to incorporate that activity into your life. If so, add a star to that activity so you can easily refer to it later to create your Thriving Plan. These activities build on each other, so try each activity on the day that it is presented to you.

This reset will only work if you are an active and committed partner in the process. You can find shelves and shelves of self-help books in stores; however, *actual changes in behavior by the readers rarely occur*. This all-too-common lack of benefit comes from books that do not teach you practical skill-building. That's exactly what we're going to do here. When you get to the second part of the book, I will ask you not only to try the activities—

all of them—but also to set reminders on your phone, or to use a visual reminder such as placing this book by your alarm clock or coffeemaker, so you see it and remember to take action. You might even want to create a reset challenge with others in your life who also live with chronic pain. Consider inviting people whom you like and trust to join you on this journey as part of your reset team. You might want to identify a prize, a desired object or experience, that you will collect after trying all the activities over the thirty days. Whatever works for you is fine by me, as long as you commit to spending at least 15 minutes a day trying and evaluating the activities, and then building and following your Thriving Plan.

Your Thriving Plan differs from most pain self-management programs because it's not only helpful but personalized and meant to be fun. Your plan will consist of activities and practices that make sense to you, work for you, and that you enjoy doing. If you don't like going to the gym, you don't have to go to the gym! How about that? You will know exactly which activities to add to your Thriving Plan because you'll have tried all thirty of them and have a good sense of which ones resonate with you.

Now, here are a few necessary caveats. This program doesn't substitute for regular medical or psychological care. Add this program to the care you already are receiving. Where the program suggests physical activity or exercise, always check with your physician to confirm that such activity is OK for you. This program is for chronic pain *not* due to cancer, although some activities and practices can help people cope with cancer pain, too. All the activities are intended to increase feelings of happiness, but some people living with chronic pain feel depressed and may need support from a mental healthcare provider. If so, please consult the Resources section in the back of this book (page 255) and seek appropriate help.

Having negative thoughts and feelings is completely normal for people living with chronic pain. Indeed, when you have chronic pain, many negative feelings are even expected. Here, I am asking you to allow those negative thoughts and feelings to exist without judgment; they are, after all, simply part of being human. But I also want you to hold space for having more positive thoughts, feelings, and experiences. You can do that, right?

In addition to me, other guides and companions will show you the road forward. In the "Lived Experience" sections throughout this book, fascinating people share their stories, reflections, and tips for living a better, more rewarding life despite living with chronic pain.

All right, are you ready to get started? If so, let's go! Take a deep cleansing breath and turn the page of this book and your life.

PART ONE

You Have the Power to Hit Reset

PAIN IS IN YOUR BRAIN

The pain you experience might have little to do with tissue or joint damage. Numerous studies have shown that some people have perfectly normal-looking X-rays or MRI scans of, say, the neck, back, or knee, but they still report intense pain in those locations. Others have scans that show obvious problems that should feel terribly painful, yet they experience no pain in those parts of their body, which I understand from personal experience.

As I sat anxiously on the exam table, the physician assistant was reviewing an MRI of my right kneecap. Bad news. "You broke it," he said.

I had never broken a bone before. Two days earlier, my boot had snagged on an all-weather floor mat at my favorite café. In slow motion, my latte flew into the air, my laptop bag followed it with considerable velocity, then *thud*—a face plant. My right knee met the tile floor with a crack and fractured.

"How's your *left* knee feel?" the PA asked, eyebrows furrowed.

My left knee? I told him that it felt fine.

"Well, you have pretty significant osteoarthritis of the left knee. The right knee isn't great either, and that likely contributed to the fracture, but your left knee . . . are you sure it doesn't hurt?"

It didn't, which I proved by moving my left leg easily in all directions.

"Huh," he said, with a look of curiosity and suspicion.

So how can this be? Blame it on the brain. The brain can amplify pain from an existing injury, nerve damage, or inflammation, or it can produce pain *completely on its own*.[1] You feel pain in your neck, back, or knee, but pain doesn't exist in that spot unless your brain interprets it to be there. Also, not just one area of your brain processes pain signals. Several areas do, and they interconnect via complex networks that involve even more areas of your brain. Think of your brain's interconnectivity like an airline map showing all the places that its planes fly. Some areas, more heavily traveled and interconnected, serve as major hubs. If you have chronic pain, your hubs are different than those of people without chronic pain.[2] It's as if you've got planes flying to the wrong destinations! That can't be good.

To complicate matters further, some of the structures, hubs, and networks of the brain that process pain overlap with the structures, hubs, and networks that process thoughts and emotions. That interconnectivity helps explain why your pain can feel so much worse when you're thinking troubling thoughts or feeling worried, stressed, or depressed. Without the brain to interpret painful sensations, pain doesn't exist. No, really. Think about a patient under general anesthesia and undergoing major surgery. The surgeon cuts a big hole in the patient's body, but they don't feel pain until they wake up in the recovery room and their brain begins processing information again. Then . . . ouch!

Your brain, to switch to a different metaphor, functions like the conductor of a symphony orchestra. An orchestra is comprised of many different musical instruments that produce a wide range of sounds. When warming up, they create a discordant jumble of hoots, thumps, and twangs. But when the conductor taps the baton on the podium, the performers come to order. A beat or two of silence follows, and then—with regular, meaningful movements of the baton that set tempo, control it, and otherwise coordinate the collective—the conductor coaxes purposeful, synchronized, beautiful music from the orchestra. At times, the performers provide feedback to the conductor, make mistakes, chit-chat with one another, or even act unruly. All of this holds true for your body, but make no mistake: The conductor (your brain) oversees and directs everything that's happening.

Before we get any further in the exploration of the brain's role in pain, something must be said. Your pain is real. Once more with feeling: *your pain is real!* What I hope to convey to you is that you also have the power to influence the pain signals traveling between your brain and body in such a way that you can make your pain better, less unpleasant, or completely go away for at least a while if not for good. When we supercharge the pain circuits in our brain with stress, fear, resentment, hopelessness, anger, and sadness we make the pain worse; however, when we choose to mix in joy, friendship, calm, love, purpose, and fun activities, we can influence the pain signals and make the pain much better.

Farm-Fresh Research

I'm a principal investigator at the Chronic Pain and Fatigue Research Center (CPFRC) in the Department of Anesthesiology at the University of Michigan. The center sits in a handsome office complex inspired by the architecture of Frank Lloyd Wright, surrounded by a farm containing a large herd of bison—seriously. Our team consists of about a dozen exceptional scientists; twenty or so program managers, study coordinators, research assistants; and student trainees who do a lot of the real work. Physician Dan Clauw, pain psychologist Dave Williams, and neuroscientist Steve Harte lead the CPFRC. I am director of pain and opioid research for the department and lead the clinical trials research team at the Back & Pain Center, our outpatient clinic.*

The nonnegotiable core principle of CPFRC research is that chronic pain is *not* a psychiatric disorder. Inferring that chronic pain is masked

---

* To learn more about our research group—including the amazing work done by each investigator, the crazy critters we see from our office windows, Bernie the groundhog, monkey-skull sessions, outrageous lunch conversations, Meat Monday, and Bye-Bye Ice Cream—check out my *Chronic Pain Reset* podcast at AftonHassett.com.

depression or hypochondria is wrong. Those antiquated ideas stand completely out of step with the neuroscience of pain. It's widely accepted that many people with chronic pain have a pain processing system in the brain that's too sensitive and reactive. It's thought that such pain sensitivity is due in part to genetic and biological factors and the rest to environmental factors that stress the brain and body, such as adverse childhood experiences, systemic racism, sexism, trauma, toxic work environments, financial stressors, infectious disease, lack of exercise, poor sleep, substance use, loneliness, and many more considerations.

Many people with pain sensitivity also have generalized sensory sensitivity, which makes them highly sensitive to bright lights, loud noises, strong odors, and potentially intense social stimuli such as strong emotions, rejection, conflict, and interpersonal violence.[3] This sensory sensitivity can worsen the side effects of medication, derailing treatment for pain and other conditions. Does any of that ring true for you, too?

The sensitized brain can have increased sensitivity to inner stimuli as well, such as your heartbeat, pulse, breathing, digestion, urge to urinate, muscle twinges, and so on. This sensitivity to activities within your body is called "interoception," a fancy word for your ability to detect and feel internal bodily processes. For all these sensitivities, the central nervous system (your brain and spinal cord) seems to be set to "high," and the brain amplifies information from both the environment and the body *with an enthusiasm unknown to mankind*, as University of Michigan football coach Jim Harbaugh might put it. When this happens, a whisper sounds like a scream, a sweet scent becomes a dizzying stench, and muscle aches can make you feel like you've been hit by a bus. Worse yet, your brain can interpret this amplified sensory information as a potential threat and activate your stress-response system, triggering an unnecessary fight-flight-or-freeze response. More about these false alarms in coming chapters.

People who have general sensory sensitivity sometimes refer to themselves as being highly sensitive persons (HSPs). Increases in scientific research and lay books and articles about life as an HSP imply a growing appreciation of this phenomenon. You're not alone if you have these types of intense sensitivities. Going forward, I'll use the term "generalized sensory sensitivity" because it describes a potentially modifiable brain process and not a problem with you as a human being.

Led by members of our team, a landmark study provided some of the first evidence of sensory sensitivity in people with chronic pain. It compared people with fibromyalgia to healthy volunteers (people without chronic pain) on tests of pain sensitivity and brain activation in response to pain. In the experiment, a device applied dull pressure to the thumb nailbed, generating moderate pain in people lying quietly in a brain scanner (fMRI). Our team found that the device had to apply almost *twice* the pressure to the nailbed of the pain-free volunteers to elicit the same verbal pain rating and similar brain activation pattern as people with chronic pain. The findings showed that the brains of people with chronic pain amplify the signal to make it feel even more painful. Since this study, many researchers have found extensive evidence of greater pain sensitivity in fibromyalgia and other chronic pain conditions, including chronic low back pain, pelvic pain, irritable bowel syndrome (IBS), temporomandibular joint pain (TMJ), migraine, osteoarthritis, rheumatoid arthritis, and others.[4]

Rewiring

The notion of sensitization comes from an old neuroscience axiom: Neurons that fire together, wire together. This adage means that the more the brain activates and processes a signal or series of signals, the more likely the brain will "remember" these signals and process them again in the same way—perhaps automatically. Think about riding a bicycle or driving a car. Even if it's been years since you steered either vehicle, you could do it again right now without much difficulty. That's your central nervous system storing automatic motor memory.

Where pain is concerned, the real estate devoted to pain processing in your brain expands (more neurons at work over larger areas in your brain), and these neurons become more sensitive and ready to fire together, thus transmitting a pain signal. Your pain becomes automatic, a bit like riding a bike. This happens because the brain has plasticity and remains pliable throughout your life. It's because of the brain's ability to rewire to process pain to excess that this type of pain is known as "nociplastic" pain.[5] *Noci* means pain in Latin, and *plastic* comes from the ancient Greek word meaning "to mold." When you have nociplastic pain, your brain has rewired itself and become very good at processing pain signals—too good. The brain can learn many unhelpful things, including how to generate pain at will, so my job is to help you help your brain learn something new and better.

A clever experiment showed just how quickly the brain can rewire itself. In a neuroimaging study led by Dillan Newbold, a team at Washington University in St. Louis, Missouri, put plaster casts on the arms of study participants for two weeks, rendering them unable to use one arm at all. The research team conducted a series of daily brain scans, 152 scans in total, to see how the volunteers' brains responded. Without regular use of that arm, rapid changes affected the motor-movement processing areas of the brain related to the immobile arm. The neurons not being used by that arm went dormant. Investigators also observed pulses of spontaneous activity in the unused brain areas that helped these dormant neurons spring back into action once the casts came off and the study participants started using their arms again. This study illustrates not only the rapid rewiring that can take place in the brain but also, importantly, that it can return to its previous state without maintenance of the processes that rewired in the first place.[6] What does that mean for you? It means that, if you want long-lasting improvement, you need to develop a program to help you maintain changes over time. You need a long-term Thriving Plan that will help your brain create new connections to buffer pain signals instead of amplifying them.

Top-Down, Bottom-Up, or Both

Another principle that might be helpful for you to understand is the idea of top-down and bottom-up pain. "Top" means the brain, while "bottom" refers to the rest of the body, neck to toes. Bottom-up pain comes from pain generators in the body, which might include inflammation from rheumatoid arthritis, bone grinding on bone in osteoarthritis, or nerve damage from an injury. In contrast, top-down pain can start in the brain and doesn't require ongoing signals from pain generators somewhere in the body.[7] Nociplastic pain is the scientific name for brain-amplified or brain-created top-down pain. Typical top-down pain conditions can include fibromyalgia, chronic low back pain, TMJ, interstitial cystitis, IBS, tension headache, chronic prostatitis, and many others. Going forward, I will mostly refer to nociplastic pain as top-down pain.

Why, you might ask, does the source matter? Pain is pain, right? Well, the most important reason is that different kinds of pain require different types of treatment. For bottom-up pain, we want to fix, if possible, whatever in the body is generating the pain. Replace the affected knee, fix the disc, decrease the inflammation in the hands, or strengthen weak muscles. If you've had painful areas of your body "fixed," such as having a knee replaced or back surgery and the pain refuses to go away, then you likely have top-down pain.

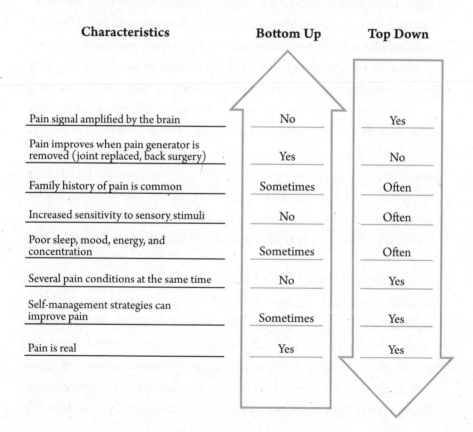

Characteristics	Bottom Up	Top Down
Pain signal amplified by the brain	No	Yes
Pain improves when pain generator is removed (joint replaced, back surgery)	Yes	No
Family history of pain is common	Sometimes	Often
Increased sensitivity to sensory stimuli	No	Often
Poor sleep, mood, energy, and concentration	Sometimes	Often
Several pain conditions at the same time	No	Yes
Self-management strategies can improve pain	Sometimes	Yes
Pain is real	Yes	Yes

The most effective approach for top-down pain is to target the brain with treatments such as medications that alter neurotransmitter concentrations or behavioral treatments that promote changes through exercise and other physical activity, changing the emotions that overlap with the pain signals, altering mindset to replace negative thoughts, and establishing new behaviors that promote well-being. All these strategies have the potential to result in functional and structural changes in your brain. The table on page 9 provides an overview of some of the characteristics of these two types of pain.

Here's another critical idea. Pain isn't binary. It doesn't have to operate as either top-down or bottom-up. Our research and that of others has shown that most people with chronic pain likely have a combination of these two types of pain, which we describe as a mixed-pain condition. In those cases, people can benefit from both treatment strategies. For example, a person with rheumatoid arthritis also might have fibromyalgia and could benefit from medications to reduce inflammation *and* medications that target pain neurotransmitters, improving quality of sleep, and engaging in enjoyable physical activities.

Please take a moment to review the summary points below. This is by far the most technical chapter in the book but the one I really want you to understand. I encourage you to read it again and highlight sections that resonate with you.

IDEAS TO REMEMBER

- The brain can amplify pain signals from the body and even generate pain completely on its own.
- Many people with heightened pain sensitivity can have generalized sensory sensitivity, making them highly sensitive to bright lights, loud noises, strong odors, medications, and potentially intense social stimuli, such as feeling rejected or scrutinized.
- Your brain can amplify pain and other sensory signals and perceive them as a physical threat, activating your stress-response system unnecessarily (like a false alarm).
- Areas of the brain that process pain signals also process thoughts and emotions in a way that negative thoughts and emotions can make pain worse and vice versa. More positive thoughts and emotions can lessen the experience of pain.
- The brain has plasticity, meaning that it can change in structure and function in a way that could help improve how you experience pain.
- Long-lasting pain improvement requires a long-term plan. By the end of this book, you'll have the tools needed to help you help your brain create and maintain new circuits that buffer pain signals instead of amplifying them.

Lived Experience: Ben

As I sat on my board waiting for the right wave, feeling the ocean rise and fall underneath me, it never occurred to me that my life was about to change radically. At age twenty-five, I was the picture of good health: strong and fit, a semiprofessional surfer, working as a corrective exercise specialist in New York City. Then came Lyme disease, and *everything* changed.

Eight years ago, I was bedbound with chronic Lyme disease for the majority of three years. I tried everything: IV infusions of antibiotics, coffee enemas, and crystal-bed therapy. Western medicine, Eastern medicine— you name it, I tried it. For years after the infection subsided, I found myself stuck in a vicious cycle of chronic pain, fatigue, anxiety, and depression. Every time I felt a bit better and tried to return to living a full life, all the old symptoms came back, and it was never clear why. Doctors didn't have the answers, so I took healing into my own hands.

A funny thing happens when you spin an egg. If you spin a raw egg, stop it from spinning, and let go again, it will resume spinning on its own because the yolk and white inside the egg are still in motion. That's how I felt during that time. I could get a handle on myself for brief moments during meditation, deep breathing, or relaxation exercises, but the moment I stepped back into the world, it was as if some internal wiring mechanism started me spinning again, just like that egg.

I told a friend that it reminded me of when I used to surf. Sometimes you end up deep underwater but can look up and see the surface, the light and blue sky above. I felt like I was stuck fifty feet underwater, and life was happening on the surface. Sometimes I could make it to the surface, but the moment I stopped struggling and kicking, I sank all the way back down. Worse yet, I felt like I had a scuba weight belt around my waist, making the struggle that much harder. I told her that I wished for a way to take off the weights and make my way to the top.

"Well, Ben," she said, "what are the weights?"

Not until I turned my attention to the brain and used neuroscience to understand what was happening did I learn that the weights were old wiring and obsolete programming in key areas of my brain. As it turns out, if you've experienced a period of long-term stress and then a powerful environmental trigger—in my case, a bacterial infection—these two events can collide to create an overactive stress response and other biological changes that Dr. Hassett discusses throughout this book. I also learned that the brain has the incredible ability to reset itself and to adapt back to normal. Some 86 billion neurons, once considered fairly static, can rewire themselves. Your brain literally can change its structure and its function, especially how your stress-response system works. The best news is that you have the power to drive this change.

After ten months of dedicated, self-directed neuroplasticity training, like what appears in this book, my symptoms completely subsided, and my health has returned fully. In a TEDx talk, I recounted that the biggest takeaway for me was that the body and mind already have all the resources that they need in order to be healthy and calm. We just need to identify and harness those resources.

Ben Ahrens is a TEDx speaker, chronic illness recovery expert, and cofounder of re-orgin.com. Learn more about his story and his science-based brain retraining program at: re-origin.com/program.

2

CO-OCCURRING SYMPTOMS
AND CONDITIONS

Before I joined the research team at the University of Michigan, I was intrigued by how Daniel Clauw, director of the Chronic Pain and Fatigue Research Center, thought about pain. In the rheumatology research world, Dan's was the dissenting voice about the underlying cause of pain conditions such as fibromyalgia and chronic low back pain. He was one of the first to suggest that the problem underlying fibromyalgia was an idiosyncrasy in how the brain processed pain (top-down) rather than a problem with muscles, as originally thought. He also proposed that these top-down, brain-driving pain processes can co-occur in other chronic pain conditions, including osteoarthritis, lupus, and rheumatoid arthritis. He emphasized that other symptoms such as fatigue, poor sleep, and difficulty concentrating accompany chronic pain and might even prove more life-altering than the pain itself. But the kicker was that Dan dared to challenge the commonly held belief that psychiatric conditions or a psychiatric disorder in disguise caused most chronic pain. In the early years, Dan's focus on a biological explanation for the pain wasn't a popular position among his colleagues.

The Ugly History of Treating Chronic Pain

Let's face it. If you have chronic pain, you likely have met a dismissive health-care professional. I'm not talking about the kind-yet-misinformed type but rather the professional who is downright unprofessional in approaching your pain and other symptoms. There you are, feeling like hell, but you dare to hope for help and yet again are disappointed by a healthcare worker's reaction. There could be a smirk involved, perhaps a curt "There's nothing really wrong with you," or the ever-irritating referral to psychiatry, which implies that your pain is purely psychological. Perhaps, after five minutes of conversation or fewer, you get a prescription for an addictive painkiller. For some, this is a godsend, but for too many those meds become a godforsaken rabbit hole that can turn destructive very quickly.

At scientific meetings, Dan has been known to confront uninformed and dismissive healthcare professionals. After most scientific talks, the speaker takes audience questions. Picture the environment. The speaker, in this case, Dan, stands at a podium, on a raised stage, with slides projected on a fifteen-by-thirty-foot screen. Lights illuminate him and the faces of the hundreds or sometimes thousands of attendees. Audience members approach the micro-phones in the seating area. After a few thoughtful questions from engaged professionals, someone invariably will approach the mic with a smug expres-sion and an air of superiority. The audience listens to this new questioner, who, in diplomatic but easy-to-decipher code words, calls pain patients whin-ers and implies that their care is a waste of physician time. All eyes dart back to Dan because those who know him know what's coming next: a weapons-grade verbal smackdown. Dan is kind and gentle with people who simply are unaware of recent scientific data or evidence, but when this lack of knowledge combines with arrogance or dismissiveness of patient suffering—well, pass the popcorn. Dan understands that it's crucial for scientists to stand up for patients. Armed with a powerful arsenal of neuroscience findings cultivated from the hard work of Rick Harris and Steve Harte, lead neuroscientists from our group and many others,[8] Dan dismantles outdated beliefs and believers with aplomb. Here are three of his most common rebuttals.

1. Chronic Pain Is Not a Psychiatric Illness

Yes, depression and anxiety commonly occur in conditions such as chronic low back pain and fibromyalgia. Upward of 50 percent of people with chronic pain have a lifetime history of depression. That rate is certainly high, but it doesn't account for 100 percent of patients, nor does it explain away the pain. As a matter of fact, close to 30 percent of people in America will have a depressive episode at some point in their lives. Get this: Lifetime rates of depression in people who suffer a heart attack are about 40 percent, but nobody's telling them that their heart attack is purely psychiatric, right?[9] If chronic pain is a psychiatric illness, then why haven't about half of people with chronic pain ever had a psychiatric illness in their lifetimes much less a current one?

A couple of recent studies conducted by our group help us understand the factors that do put people at risk for chronic pain. Chelsea Kaplan and Andrew Schrepf, two brilliant young researchers from our team, showed, in an elegant pair of studies that followed children over several years, that depression and anxiety didn't increase the risk that a child would develop widespread chronic pain later in life. Instead, having poor sleep, numerous bodily symptoms, cognitive problems (difficulty with concentration, attention), and *distinct changes in the structure and the function of the brain* predicted which children later developed chronic pain. These data suggest that depression and anxiety don't come before pain nor do they predict its onset.[10]

2. Symptoms in Addition to Chronic Pain Don't Mean That the Patient Is Exaggerating

As noted earlier, five symptoms tend to occur together in people with pain. When you have a cold, symptoms such as coughing, runny nose, headache, fatigue, difficulty concentrating, and feeling blah (cranky or apathetic) co-occur. In chronic pain, other symptoms often include poor sleep, fatigue, difficulty concentrating, and feeling blah (poor mood). Notice a pattern? When you're unwell, such as when you have a cold or flu, you feel tired, are in a bad mood, and can't think straight. The brilliant design of your immune system makes that happen.

When a virus or bacterium infects you, your immune system kicks into high gear and releases cytokines, the immune system's communication team and strike force, which seek and destroy invaders. Cytokines usually trigger inflammation, a sure sign that your body is trying to kill unwanted guests. The release of certain types of cytokines, commonly called sickness cytokines, also explains why you feel so lousy when you get sick. This behavioral aspect of your immune response can help you survive (retire to a cave so a giant predator doesn't eat you) and helps you not spread disease to the rest of your tribe. So, yes, symptoms cluster in a predictable manner, and their manifestation and expression can serve an important purpose. Unfortunately, these overlapping symptoms can make you feel much worse than having just pain alone. But there's some good news coming in a bit.

3. Having Multiple Chronic Pain Conditions and Seeing Many Specialists Doesn't Make the Patient a Hypochondriac

The medical community often fails to see the bigger picture. You likely have heard the old parable that has roots in ancient India. A group of blind men encounters an elephant for the first time and tries to figure it out based on what they can feel with their hands. Each man reaches out and touches a different part of the elephant's body and describes what he understands. The man who touches a leg thinks they've found a new type of tree. Another man, who finds the trunk, is sure it's a powerful snake. Each is certain that what he knows is true, unwilling to consider the broader picture. Some of these men even become enraged, believing that the other men must be lying because the answer is so obvious. In some versions of the story, the disagreements end in bloodshed. The moral of the story is that we humans tend to believe that, based on our subjective and limited experience, we alone possess the truth.

This tendency helps explain why each subspecialty in medicine has its own unique chronic pain condition. In rheumatology, which considers the whole body and all systems, fibromyalgia commonly is diagnosed. In orthopedics, chronic low back pain is thought to explain away the pain, while in dentistry, the pain is attributed to temporomandibular disorder (jaw pain). In many cases, a physician diagnosing pain in the lower back doesn't ask about more widespread pain, such as fibromyalgia. Similarly, the doctor who diagnoses fibromyalgia might not ask about IBS (pain in the gut) or chronic headaches. Consequently, people with chronic pain often accumulate several diagnoses because they see different physicians who each make a diagnosis based on the body part they know and love. Unfortunately, this scattershot approach misses the big picture. It's an elephant!

Chronic pain conditions are complex; they upend lives, and a respectful approach is required. As the neuroscience of pain slowly makes its way into day-to-day medical practice, Dan's firm push-back of physicians and researchers with antiquated ideas is required less and less, which is reassuring. Still, most medical trainees don't receive adequate education about causes and the need for interdisciplinary and more comprehensive pain care. It's also important for healthcare providers not to lose sight of the humans and the human potential that sit atop that exam table, feeling vulnerable and looking for help.

When we teach new healthcare trainees about diseases and conditions, it's often helpful to share a case to make the symptoms and disease concepts come alive. Kindly indulge my desire to do the same for you. This is the case of a forty-four-year-old Caucasian male who has severe chronic low back pain. It began in college, likely from a football injury. Since those early years, he has undergone multiple back surgeries, none resulting in adequate relief. The most recent surgery was complicated by sepsis, a full-body infection so severe that it nearly killed him. Over the years, he has sought treatment from many physicians and other healthcare professionals, and he is taking multiple pain and other medications. Yet his severe pain persists, at times completely disabling. Several specialists all see his pain as arising from different causes and emanating from different parts of the body. He is seeing an orthopedist (spine), urologist (prostate), otolaryngologist (ear, nose, and throat), and endocrinologist (Addison's disease). He has been diagnosed with several chronic pain conditions throughout his life, including IBS, which began in childhood, and in adulthood: chronic prostatitis, chronic low back pain, headache, and myofascial pain (widespread pain). He also has a history of insomnia and depression. His IBS symptoms are severe enough at times to cause total incapacitation yet aren't as disruptive as the low back pain, which plagues him daily.

Aspects of this case might feel quite familiar. Unfortunately, it wouldn't be unheard of for a physician reviewing this case to think regretfully: *lost cause*. You might sense the same hopelessness for the man in the case study or perhaps in your own life. But what if I told you that the patient in this case was President John F. Kennedy? Does that change anything? What do his remarkable achievements and lasting influence on American and global history say about the power of resiliency? You still can lead a meaningful, influential, and productive life despite living with chronic illness and pain.[11]

SPACE: The Final Frontier

So what about all those co-occurring symptoms that complicate life with chronic pain? Another colleague and friend from the CPFRC whom I want you to know is David Williams. Dave is a fellow psychologist, pain researcher, and a talented musician. Based on his work over the years, he created the acronym SPACE to refer to a cluster of symptoms in chronic pain:

Sleep
Pain
Affect (anxiety, depression, malaise)
Cognition (poor concentration or clarity of thought, memory issues, brain fog)
Energy (fatigue)[12]

Dave and other members from our team, including Andrew Schrepf and Steve Harte, have led efforts to show that these symptoms all interconnect, likely the product of a combination of widespread and excessive sensitivity within the central nervous system and/or persistent low-level inflammation throughout the body.

Each person experiences a unique SPACE symptom pattern. Some might have all the symptoms equally. For others, one symptom rises above the rest, and the most disruptive symptom isn't always pain. I once conducted a study in which Elizabeth Hale, a colleague from Britain, helped me interview people with lupus to learn more about their pain and how living with the disease affected their self-image. We found that the disease did damage their self-image and body image and that, counter to our hypothesis, fatigue was by far the most soul-crushing symptom for them, not pain.[13]

What SPACE symptoms do you experience? If you like, make a list. These symptoms tend to fluctuate over time, but which symptom generally troubles you the most? What, if anything, can you do right now to make that symptom better? You might have more luck addressing your pain by sneaking up on it by improving another symptom. This approach acts sort of like a secret weapon. (Shh, don't tell your pain.)

Here's how it works. Let's say pain is your worst symptom, and you can't do much to find relief. You're a "good patient" and generally follow doctor's orders. You eat well, get a bit of exercise daily, but still the pain persists. Maybe your other significant SPACE symptoms are sleep and affect (depressive symptoms). Here's how you execute a sneak attack on the pain. If you improve your sleep, you likely will find that your pain and mood improve, too. The same goes for improving your mood. Inject a little more happiness into your day, and you likely will sleep better and, in turn, experience less pain. When you sleep better and feel happier, you tend to engage in more enjoyable activities and generally get more exercise. We know this strategy works because study participants have worn activity monitors (like fancy fitness trackers) and rated their symptoms throughout the day and over time. Over and over, we see clear patterns of symptom change in relationship to other symptom change. Better mood leads to better sleep; better sleep results in less fatigue; less fatigue makes concentration easier; and better mood and sleep result in less pain. The combinations are many, but the results are the same. Your physical and mental well-being can improve if you improve even just one of these symptoms.

Let's take stock of your SPACE profile. Rank how bothersome each

symptom feels to you. The most bothersome symptom gets a 1, and the
least bothersome symptom gets a 5.

_____ **Sleep**

_____ **Pain**

_____ **Affect** (anxiety, depression, malaise)

_____ **Cognition** (poor concentration or clarity of thought,
memory issues, brain fog)

_____ **Energy** (fatigue)

SPACE symptoms can respond well to many of the activities you'll be
trying in part two of this book, and your SPACE profile will help guide you
as you explore them and then develop your Thriving Plan. In the mean-
time, start plotting your sneak-attack strategy to defeat your pain, such as
improving your sleep, exercise habits, or emotional well-being. Your pain
won't see it coming!

IDEAS TO REMEMBER

- Chronic pain isn't a psychiatric illness; however, living with
  chronic pain can result in psychiatric illness. Depression, anxiety, stress, and trauma are common in people with chronic pain,
  just as in most medical diseases and illnesses.
- Top-down pain conditions overlap with one another (for
  example, fibromyalgia and IBS), and they also overlap with
  inflammatory and mechanical pain conditions (rheumatoid
  arthritis, osteoarthritis).
- SPACE stands for sleep, pain, affect, cognition, and energy and
  refers to symptoms that commonly cluster when people have
  illnesses.
- You can perform a sneak-attack on your pain by improving
  other symptoms, such as poor sleep or anxiety and depression.

3

STRESS AND THE PRICE
THE BODY PAYS

No researcher accomplishes anything without a competent and invested team. I have the best team anywhere, led by Sana Shaikh, my uber-amazing program coordinator. Sana earned an MD but has chosen a high-level career in research-study oversight. (I'm *so* lucky to have her.) About a year after completing medical school, her sister, a psychologist, was discussing with her the extreme stress that she observed Sana experiencing during medical school.

"That was *stress*?" Sana said. "I thought I just had a lot to do and had to figure out how to get everything done like everyone else."

"Seriously?" her sister replied. "You weren't aware that you were completely stressed out? I was so concerned."

Sana thought about that period of her life from a different perspective and wondered, *Could this really be true?* She then remembered a night during her third year of medical school when her fiancé called and all she could do was sob and gasp into the phone.

"Honey, please tell me what's wrong," he begged her.

She finally put her finger on the source of her excruciating misery. Instead of an upcoming exam or the unrelenting stress of medical school, she uttered between sobs and sniffles: *"The sink . . . is full . . . of dishes!"*

Even if we fail to recognize it or its many sources, stress is powerful, all-consuming, and an undeniable part of our lives. People often ask me about the role stress plays in chronic pain. It plays many roles not just in chronic pain but in most human diseases and illnesses.[14] First, it can trigger the onset of disease in already vulnerable people. Persistent stress over time also can result in physiological changes in the brain and body that set the stage for the development of many medical illnesses, not just chronic pain. Such changes can include the disruption of a healthy stress-response system, as well as the immune system. Lastly, stress damages our health behaviors, meaning what we do generally to take care of ourselves. For example, stressed people are less likely to sleep well, eat healthy food, exercise, take time to relax, socialize with friends, and follow doctor recommendations.

Because stress is so pivotal and can impact your pain on multiple levels, many of the strategies you will learn and try are designed to help you better cope with stress. Improving how you react to the inevitably craptastic parts of life has the potential to change your quality of life and overall health radically. Let's explore three roles that stress can play in human health, followed by what you can do about it.

Role 1: Stress Pulls the Trigger

The vulnerability-stress model of human health and illness proposes that most diseases and conditions result from a combination of genetic factors (vulnerability) and environmental factors (triggers) that set the disease process in motion. Diseases and conditions that fit into this category are called multifactorial genetic inheritance disorders (this will not be on the quiz) and include heart disease, high blood pressure, diabetes, cancer, obesity, and arthritis. This list of conditions accounts for most of the chronic health problems afflicting humanity. Most top-down pain conditions fall into this same category.

Numerous studies tell us that a genetic vulnerability for chronic pain is likely. For example, family studies show that people with chronic pain often have first-degree biological relatives who have chronic pain, too.[15] Other studies have shown that a wide array of genetic mutations could underlie a vulnerability for chronic pain.[16] For the environmental part, it's also common for people with chronic pain to report a triggering event that happened right before the pain started. Such environmental stressors or triggers can include physical trauma (car accident, broken bone, surgery), psychological trauma (emotional abuse, a life-threatening event, major loss), infectious disease (more about that later), or persistent daily stress (toxic family, dangerous commute, miserable job). Chronic pain often begins with a genetic vulnerability that one or a combination of those powerful environmental stressors can trigger.

Role 2: Your Body Pays the Price

Let's begin with understanding that your stress-response system is a good thing. Like just about everything else related to body and mind, it originates in the brain and has a purpose. When you detect a potential threat in the environment (*"OMG, a snake!"*), your amygdala—a primitive structure in your brain that processes emotion—activates. The activated amygdala blares a feverish alarm (*threat!*) to your hypothalamus, your brain's command center. The hypothalamus initiates the fight-flight-or-freeze response, which includes activating your sympathetic nervous system, a fancy phrase for your bodily freak-out system. As if flooring the gas pedal of a car, your sympathetic nervous system immediately makes your heart race, breathing quicken, pupils dilate, mouth dry, skin tingle, digestion slow, and your immune system prepare for possible injury. Adrenaline and other stress messengers pump furiously throughout your body to promote lightning-fast action. In a matter of milliseconds, you become ready to respond to the threat.

Once the threat has passed (*"Hahaha, just a garden hose. Phew!"*), the *para*sympathetic nervous system slows everything back down. It reverses all the physiological changes initiated by the sympathetic nervous system. Your body goes back to normal, and balance is restored. When the para-

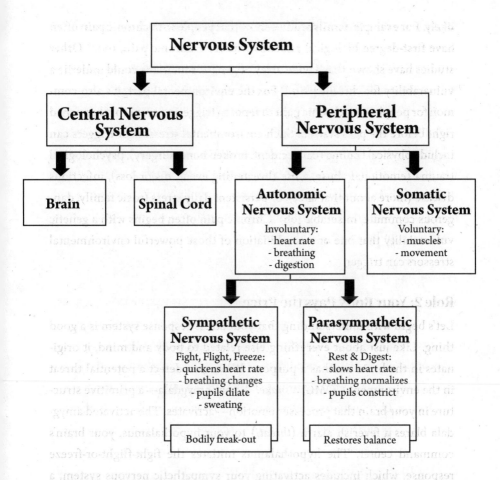

sympathetic nervous system activates, you generally feel relaxed, at peace, perhaps even ready for a nap. The diagram above shows a simplified version of the divisions of labor for your nervous system.

Disrupting a Healthy Stress-Response System

Many people with chronic pain have a sympathetic nervous system activated too easily and often persistently, as if they're living in fight-flight-or-freeze mode most of the time. Why? Blame it on the false alarms. The fight-flight-or-freeze system kicks into gear to save you from threats. The problem for us modern humans is that the brain interprets many stressful situations that aren't life-threatening as life-threatening. The body doesn't know the difference. Then, for people with chronic pain, the pain signal itself can be perceived as a near-constant or constant threat. Not helpful! Other typically nonthreatening stimuli such as loud noises, strong smells, and even negative social interactions can be interpreted as threats, too.

If false alarms that lead to perpetual fight, flight, or freeze aren't a big enough problem, people with chronic pain often have difficulty reestablishing balance. Their parasympathetic nervous systems struggle to calm everything back down. The good news is that many simple relaxation techniques can help you dial down those engine-revving bodily freakouts and help you strengthen your calming parasympathetic nervous system, thus resetting your balance back to normal.

Disrupting the Immune System

When your body exists in fight-flight-or-freeze mode too much of the time, it faces immune system consequences, too. The stress-response system and immune system constantly communicate. If the stress-response system continuously blares *"Emergency!"* the immune system responds in several ways. It decreases production of antibodies to fight infectious diseases effectively. That response helps explain why, when you're very stressed, you're more prone to catching a cold, the flu, and other infectious diseases. The immune system also responds to excessive stress by producing chronic low-level inflammation throughout your body. That's not good for you because that kind of inflammation is associated with heart disease, autoimmune disease, depression, cognitive decline (including dementia), type 1 diabetes, cancer, and—you guessed it!—chronic pain.

But the plot thickens. A wide array of viruses and bacteria can precede the development of new chronic pain as well, including Epstein-Barr virus, herpesvirus, viruses that cause stomach flu, hepatitis B and C, and tickborne viruses. In almost every type of infectious disease, about 5 to 15 percent of people affected report persistent symptoms long after the infection resolves. Long COVID might fall into this same category.[17]

The exact reason that new top-down pain and other symptoms such as fatigue, malaise, brain fog, and poor sleep often follow infectious disease isn't entirely clear. The leading theory points to low-level inflammation. It's thought that some viruses result in subdued but lingering immune-system activation that lasts for months or even years. Think of the immune system, in this case, like a pot of water simmering but never reaching a rolling boil. When the immune system activates, even at a low level, cytokines (immune messengers) circulate throughout the body and cause chronic inflammation and sickness behaviors, including lethargy, withdrawal, loss of joy, and anxiousness.

Remember, sickness behaviors serve a critical survival function. They keep you in bed, away from others, and help you recover.[18] The immune system's release of sickness cytokines might help explain why people with chronic pain often feel exhausted, unmotivated, uninterested, unsocial, and just plain lousy. Obesity, poor sleep, and even persistent or toxic stress also can bring on these immune system changes, including low-level inflammation and the release of sickness cytokines. More about that below.

Role 3: Different Types of Stress Have Different Potential Health Effects

So far, we've focused on the perils of stress, but not all stress is bad. Bruce McEwen, a highly respected scientist, dedicated his life's work to shedding light on the biological foundation for how stress affects the brain and body, all the way down to the cellular level. A mentor and friend, Bruce authored nearly 1,000 research articles. His pioneering work at Rockefeller University helped the scientific community understand some of the concepts we've been discussing in this chapter. In *The End of Stress as We Know It*, he explained that we generally experience three different types of stress and each type of stress has physiological and behavioral processes associated with it.[19]

Good, Normal Stress

This kind of stress occurs when you face a challenge and succeed. Examples include winning a contest, crushing a work presentation or job interview, and planning and having a wedding.

For these events, the stress-response system activates, releasing the stress hormone cortisol. In this context, cortisol serves an adaptive function. It helps you rally for the challenge, raising you to your best. Your stress-response system also releases cortisol when you encounter everyday stressors such as a traffic jam, a work deadline, or quarreling kids. Once the event passes, your parasympathetic nervous system quiets everything back down, thus restoring balance. With good, normal stress, you experience few changes to your general health routine. In other words, your diet, exercise, and sleep patterns don't change all that much.

Tolerable Stress

This kind of stress occurs when adversity strikes, as with a painful breakup, the loss of a job, or a loved one dying. Something bad happens, but you have the personal resources you need to recover over time. Those resources consist mostly of having loving and supportive family and friends and good coping skills with which you can feel and name normal emotions, process the setback, and perhaps even find meaning or new purpose in the context of the event. With tolerable stress, the stress-response system activates and might remain activated for a while, perhaps a long while. Here, the negative effects could manifest as gaining weight or elevated blood pressure. After the worst has passed, you find your way forward again, your stress-response system quiets back down, and you return to normal, which includes maintaining your typical health routines. With this kind of stress, the goal is to be resilient to the negative effects so you can bounce back to your prior steady state.

Toxic Stress

The third type of stress happens when something terrible takes place and you don't have the personal resources (adequate healthy coping and social support) needed to bounce back. Experiencing traumatic events earlier in life might make you more vulnerable to toxic stress. Adverse childhood experiences can impair how your stress-response system functions in adulthood. With toxic stress, you might feel like you have no control (helpless) and see no path forward (hopeless). Emotionally you are vulnerable to depression and anxiety, and physiologically your body's stress-response system stays in high gear, revving that engine all the way to the red line. When you feel this awful, good health behaviors tend to disappear. Bad eating habits, lack of exercise, poor sleep, skipping medication, and avoiding doctors all can arise and put you at high risk for new or worsening diseases and conditions such as chronic pain.

Stress is part of everyday life. Not all stress is bad, and some stress even can help us perform better and succeed. Wanting or trying to avoid all stress is very stressful. Here's the deal. It's only when we have too much stress with inadequate coping skills or time for recovery that we show signs of what Bruce McEwen called allostatic load (stress-induced wear and tear on the body and brain). The key to remaining resilient is to recognize when stress has turned toxic and to strengthen the tools you need to regain balance in mind and body.

For your Thriving Plan, you need to understand the types and sources of stress in your life. Then identify, learn, and practice at least three stress-busting techniques to keep stress from becoming toxic.

Think about the stressors in your life. Make a list and categorize them as good, normal; tolerable; and toxic. Everyone's lists will look different. A stressor for one person could be a source of great fun for someone else. Next, think about how you cope (or don't cope) with each of the stressors you listed. Consider the following questions.

1. Can you identify the aspects of the stressor that you can control and do something about?
2. Do you reach out to friends or family for support? They don't need to solve the problem for you, but they can help you share the burden and brainstorm solutions.

3. Does the stressor seem so overwhelming that you (want to) blunt its effects with unhelpful behaviors, such as eating junk food or substance use/abuse?

4. When feeling intense stress, do you take care of yourself? Remember, when stressed, we tend to skip activities and behaviors that support good health: regular exercise, eating healthily, sleeping adequately, or making time for relaxation and fun.

Here's the bottom line. Every choice you make about how to cope with stress has consequences that might enhance your health or make it worse. Part Two of this book contains lots of skills and strategies aimed specifically at making you healthier and more resilient. Each daily activity is a potential stress buster, so take note of those that you think might work for your unique experience of stress.

IDEAS TO REMEMBER

- Different types of stress range from good, healthy stress to problematic, toxic stress. The types and persistence of stress have different consequences for your physical and psychological health.
- While your stress likely didn't cause your chronic pain, it probably is making your pain a lot worse.
- For many with chronic pain, "false alarms" activate the stress-response system too often.
- Constant stress-response system activation has immune system consequences, making you more vulnerable to disease and illness.
- Stressed people don't sleep well, tend to eat poorly and exercise less, and are more prone to depression and anxiety.
- Learning skills and techniques to help you cope with stress better is the key to a happier life and less pain.

Lived Experience: Cassandra

The teacher asked me to sit on a cushion on the floor. With the pain throbbing in my body, I felt skeptical that I could do that. As if reading my thoughts, he suggested that I could sit up against the wall to support my back. Well, OK, then. I was willing to try.

I had journeyed to this beautiful place to learn meditation and to practice yoga. When I first got sick, only yoga alleviated my symptoms, but I'd never meditated before. I didn't really believe any nirvana existed or that I could make my mind blank. The pain was too preoccupying. Over nine months, I had tried dozens of different medications, and nothing worked for me, or the side effects were too strong and just as disabling as the pain I was trying to escape. Yet during one of those sessions of meditation, my pain evaporated, and I was gobsmacked.

The ten days on this retreat gave me agency over my body that I hadn't had in more than two years. I experienced a sense of relief that made me hopeful that I could salvage some semblance of a life, a life that had been decimated because of my condition. Even hope had become too painful. While there, I learned how food could be medicine (or poison), how to re-inhabit the body that betrayed me, how to cultivate deep rest, and how to maintain mindfulness while flooded with pain. I came to view my relationship with my illness as a dance rather than a fight, because the metaphor of war on disease (and the use of painkillers) meant that I was always the loser. I figured out how to feel safe enough so I could call a cease-fire because, by definition, a chronic illness doesn't go away.

Because of these powerful experiences over those days, I became a yoga therapist. When I teach inversions, such as headstands or handstands, I talk about how we dance with gravity. Gravity is a given, neither good nor bad. I prefer to view my illness like gravity, a given with which I was learning to dance. After more than two decades, I became a more skillful dancer. I've learned how meditation could shift the pain. I learned how to befriend my body, accept the discomfort, and not flee it. I gingerly explored awareness of the sensations and pain and can do so with curiosity and not judgment.

At the onset of my illness, I was like a toddler learning to walk in my new world. Then I was a young child, and I was confused, asked questions, and felt that I still didn't understand so much. After I realized that I would be living with this condition for the rest of my life, I felt the anger and defiance of a teenager. What was I going to do? What could I do? What kind of pain could dissipate when I sat still and breathed deeply? It didn't happen all the time, but that it could happen and did happen empowered me.

So I'd do nothing, just hang on. I wouldn't fight gravity. I wouldn't be afraid of my feelings. I'd scream as loud as I needed and cry as hard as I must. I knew weeks of knifing pain that made me a zombie, trembling times of impossible nausea due to my pain medication, and infuriating episodes of fatigue that imprisoned me in bed. But as difficult and prolonged as those moments were, they were still only moments that would pass.

I would just hang on and extend the moment long enough for some light to creep in. That's what meditation taught me. I realized that I had experience and perspective I didn't have before. I was past the adolescent stage. I knew that it could get better, that it would get better, and eventually it did. The pas de deux finally taught me that.

Cassandra Metzger is the founder of Premier Wellness Travel. Learn more at PremierWellnessTravel.com.

4

THOUGHTS ARE BRAIN ACTIVITIES

Your thoughts hold the key to *everything*. So far, we've explored how the brain acts like the conductor of the complex orchestra that is your body. How you feel and what you do mostly come from signals originating in your brain. We next explored the effects of persistent stress and how it may not have caused your pain or other symptoms but still has the power to make them worse. Now, putting this all together in a way that can improve your health and well-being, we turn to the notion that your thoughts represent the most important tool you have for improving your experience of pain *and* your life. If you take only one point from this book—and I hope that you take it and many more—please internalize this idea:

Your thoughts about a bad event matter more
to your health than the event itself.

You can't control events; you can't control other people; but you can change how you think about them, how you react to them, and how much power you relinquish to them. Moving forward successfully requires knowing and accepting what lies beyond your control and committing to the actions, people, and goals that enrich your life. Living life in accordance with your values begins with your thoughts.

What's a Thought, Anyway?

Good question! Even with the most brilliant minds studying brain structure and function, we still don't understand fully how the brain forms thoughts or even the true nature of the mind or consciousness. We do know that, when we think, certain areas of the brain activate. Also, different and predictable areas of the brain activate when we think specific types of thoughts. For example, brain activation patterns for happy thoughts look different than patterns for sad or fearful thoughts. The part of this puzzle that matters most for people with chronic pain is that the content of our thoughts relates to how we perceive and react to physical pain. Some thoughts decrease the experience of pain, while others increase pain severity, suffering, and disability.

Thoughts Lead to Emotional, Behavioral, and Physiological Reactions

In writing this book, I pondered whether to place the chapter about emotions before the chapter discussing thoughts. Evolutionarily, emotions come first. The emotion-processing areas of the brain are ancient, existing in the brains of our ancestors long before reason and judgment. Plus, the emotion centers of the brain influence much of our behavior. Emotion-processing areas and circuitry in your brain often overlap with pain-processing areas and circuitry. Still, many principles and techniques in this book come from cognitive-behavioral therapy (CBT). In CBT, when we talk about temporal order (what comes before what) and causality (what causes what), thoughts come first.

Possibly the most widely practiced type of therapy for pain, depression, anxiety, substance use, trauma, eating disorders, and so on, CBT shows the best scientific evidence for effectiveness. It stands on the premise that our thoughts lie at the center of our suffering *and* our flourishing. How and what you think about something dictates how you react to it. Your reactions can be emotional, behavioral, and physiological, and these reactions can interact with one another. For example, your anger (emotional reaction) about another failure (negative thoughts) can make you yell at the dog (behavior), causing a racing heartbeat and muscle tension (physiological response). Then you feel bad about yelling at the dog, and your muscle tension worsens, as does your pain. *I'm such an idiot. I've triggered a flare,* you think, and now you feel sad and guilty because the dog already forgave you, but you are miles away from forgiving yourself. Sheesh.

The example above shows the importance of this process for people with chronic pain. Your ever-evolving thoughts, emotions, behavior, and physiological responses all affect your experience of pain (see figure below).

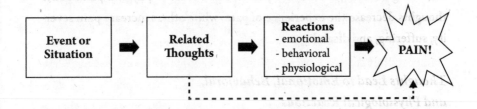

All this reacting takes place in or is initiated by your brain. The good news is that research already has shown us that CBT can help normalize pain-related brain responses in people with chronic pain by changing overly negative thought patterns.[20] Once again, your thoughts lie at the center of everything; they serve as the keystone.

Let's explore a painful social encounter, another example of how negative thoughts can influence emotions and behavior. A friend says something hurtful. Regardless of whether she intended to hurt you, you feel devastated. You wonder if there's truth to what she said. You worry whether others see you in the same negative light. You fret over your own fears about who you are and how your friends—and *everybody*—view you. Like dark thunderclouds rolling over the horizon, unhelpful thoughts emerge: *Who* *would want to be my friend anyway? I'm not lovable. I'm going to be that lonely old person with thirty-two cats!**

Negative thoughts like these make you feel even more depressed and anxious. They can disrupt your sleep, make you less likely to exercise, and compel you to eat junk food to soothe your tortured soul. Then you feel worse about yourself, irritable from too little sleep, and—oh yeah— you have chronic pain so now that is flaring, too. In the long run, feeling lousy can result in avoiding friends and other social situations. Avoidance behavior that springs from fear and anxiety sets the stage for a self-fulfilling prophecy in which you find yourself alone. Worrisome thoughts and fears make you behave in ways that make exactly what you hope to avoid *more likely to happen.*

How might the situation have differed if you sought explanations other than that you're a bad person unworthy of love? Maybe your friend was having a bad day and unintentionally lashed out at you. She might call later, asking for forgiveness, and all your worry would have been for nothing. Another solution: Rather than stewing all night, you could text her to find out what's going on. She also might not be a good friend and has made hurtful statements on other occasions without remorse. You can't control her behavior, but you can control whether she remains your friend. Perhaps, on dispassionate examination, you detect a shred of truth in what she said, and she landed on a behavior you want to change and improve. Imperfection doesn't make you unlovable—quite the opposite! Ideally, we all follow a path that allows us to change and grow. As they say: progress, not perfection. When your thoughts remain flexible and your interpretation of events more dispassionate and scientific, you open the door to new possibilities that often involve less sadness, worry, sleep loss, junk food, and pain.

Unhelpful Thoughts and Our Reactions

We all have them. They spring into action like runners at the starting line of a race. The pistol sounds (a negative event takes place) and they're off! *This*

---

* Cats are glorious creatures, but that's a *lot* of cats.

is terrible. I can't handle it. They'll think I'm [dumb, incompetent, unprepared, untalented]. These unhelpful thoughts usually come automatically. They just pop into your head. Negative, automatic thoughts like these often were programmed into your brain when you were a child, and they reside there still, waiting for the right situation to reassert themselves and mess up your day. Many of these automatic thoughts are what we call cognitive errors, and they almost always spark strong negative emotions and maladaptive behaviors. They're errors because they don't have a basis in reality, and, more than anything, *they aren't helpful!*

Unhelpful automatic thoughts usually result in unhelpful behavior: poor choices, bad actions, or a problematic lack of action such as avoidance and procrastination. For many people, negative thoughts lie at the heart of the incessant word storm that takes place in the mind, promotes excessive stress, and blocks accomplishment and contentment. Often these thoughts resulted from negative interactions between you as a child and a misguided adult. Some thoughts might have been adaptive at the time, meaning that they helped back then, but they have since grown antiquated and counterproductive. Now it's your job to recognize these thoughts as unhelpful, stare them down, step over them, and take actions that help you create a rich and meaningful life. That's what this book is all about!

In *Chatter*, his aptly titled book, Ethan Kross, a professor of psychology and researcher at the University of Michigan, discusses this phenomenon of inner dialogue and helpful solutions.[21] Self-reflection and listening to your inner voice represent an important part of emotional exploration and growth, but the chatter from your inner critic can undermine everything. Negative self-talk usually makes you narrow your focus to unimportant details, to the detriment of the bigger picture, and it can cause a lot of rumination and worry.

So how do you quiet your inner critic? It's tempting to ignore chatter completely, but it's more effective to consider the content of your thoughts with some psychological distance. Step back from the emotional entanglements and consider your thoughts in the third person as a scientist would, using curiosity and objectivity. Are these thoughts true? Are they helpful? Counseling yourself about your chatter, your inner critic, as you would counsel a friend, makes for an excellent approach. In these moments, we benefit from self-compassion. If you broaden your perspective, treat yourself with love and respect, as you would your closest friends, and set aside negative emotions and irrational thoughts, the answers sometimes become obvious.

You live with chronic pain. You probably have quite a commentary about yourself and your pain going on in your head at any time. Step back and try to gain a little perspective. How do you think of your pain? Is it a part of you but not all of you or perhaps an unwelcome invader that you battle daily? Is your pain a brutal dictator trying to overtake your life or an old, cantankerous friend that you don't really like but gives your life order and meaning? Have you ever thought about what your pain is trying to tell you? Do you ever think, *Why me?* Have you ever considered learning how to dance with your pain as Cassandra described in her story before this chapter? Your thoughts about your pain matter. Once you name and understand them, you will have much more power over your pain and how you live your life.

The best-studied type of unhelpful pain-related thought is pain "catastrophizing." We all can feel frustrated by the seeming powerlessness to do anything about unremitting, life-stealing pain. But catastrophic thoughts about your pain lead to feelings of hopelessness and helplessness that promote depression, loss of function, and even more severe pain. Examples of catastrophic thoughts include: *My pain is awful, and it's never going to get better. There's nothing I can do to improve my pain. The pain has ruined my life.* Does that sound familiar? If so, it's OK. At this point in our journey, I ask you to be objective, like a scientist, without emotion and judgment. Just increase your awareness of these thoughts. Write them down and determine whether those thoughts support your values and goals or get in the way.

Pain catastrophizing is common and therefore well-studied. As such, we know a bit about how this pattern of negative thinking relates to changes in the brain. Studies show an association between catastrophizing and changes in brain structure (gray matter thickness), neural network connectivity, and activation of brain areas involved in pain, thought, and emotional processing.[22] More specifically, it looks like catastrophizing influences pain perception by increasing the anticipation of and attention to pain. This heightened threat-seeking state sparks strong negative emotional responses often followed by unhelpful behavior. Imagine thinking that your pain is awful and never will improve. Now imagine how that thought could impact your willingness to go to physical therapy, exercise, or try a new self-management approach. You likely would think, *Why bother?*

Another common thought with chronic pain is avoidance: *If I do that, it'll hurt, so I'm not even going to try.* Many chronic pain conditions often begin with a physical injury that has long since resolved, but the pain transformed from bottom-up pain (initially due to the injury) to top-down pain (brain is now driving the pain). You and your brain are pretty darn certain that a recommended activity or exercise will cause reinjury, so you simply don't do it. At some level, you might recognize this thought as irrational, but why risk it? So, you avoid the very exercise or activity that could help you recover or lead a more rewarding life for fear that it could worsen your pain. Does that sound familiar? If so, make a note: *pain avoidance= not helpful.*

The success of CBT for treating many diseases and conditions has inspired several second-generation approaches, such as mindfulness-based stress reduction (MBSR), acceptance and commitment therapy (ACT), positive psychology, dialectical behavioral therapy (DBT), and emotion-focused CBT for pain. You will learn techniques from each of these approaches to behavioral pain care.

The Beauty of Pragmatic Optimism

As many as 80 percent of US Army soldiers return from deployment with chronic pain. We conducted a study to explore whether certain thoughts and beliefs might be protective. When deployed abroad, soldiers often experience extreme hardships, such as extended separation from loved ones, inhospitable living conditions, or combat-related injury and trauma. We tracked more than 27,000 soldiers over multiple deployments and found something surprising.[23] The soldiers' level of optimism *before* deployment greatly reduced the odds of returning with chronic pain. Despite engaging in direct combat, experiencing traumatic events such as an IED blast, seeing comrades fall, or sustaining injury themselves, optimism appeared to protect them from developing chronic pain. This finding offers a powerful example of how thoughts and mindset can impact the experience of pain.

Final Thoughts about Thoughts

Of course, we do not want to be foolish optimists; the type of person who acts recklessly, believing that no harm exists. Instead, the scientific data suggest that you remain wary of having too much optimism; inevitably life goes sideways at some point. Author, lecturer, and consultant Denis Waitley has put forward a wiser approach: "Expect the best, plan for the worst, and prepare to be surprised."

IDEAS TO REMEMBER

- Thoughts drive emotions, and thoughts and emotions dictate your behavior. Your thoughts about events, good or bad, matter more to your happiness and health than the events themselves.
- You can't change negative circumstances, events, or people, but you can change what you think about them and how you react to them.
- Self-critical automatic thoughts often come from experiences in youth. These cognitive errors or negative thoughts (catastrophizing) just pop into your head. Often, they have no basis in reality, and, more than anything, they aren't helpful.
- Most humans are wired to have a negativity bias—being watchful for potential threats might help you survive. Yet, overly negative thoughts usually result in bad actions, inaction, and poor emotional and physical well-being.
- Use a little self-compassion to quiet negative chatter coming from your inner critic who judges all your failures harshly and discounts your successes. Talk to yourself like you would talk to your closest friend: with kindness, love, and respect.
- Dare to have at least a little pragmatic optimism.

5

EMOTIONS ARE
PHYSIOLOGICAL EVENTS

For people with chronic pain, negative emotions such as depression, anxiety, anger, guilt, regret, and fear are common. It's perfectly normal to feel all these emotions. The problem arises when you repress them or allow them to fester for days, weeks, months, or years. In those cases, they can take a remarkable toll on your health and well-being. Under the influence of negative emotions, people tend to sleep worse, eat poorly, get less exercise, abuse substances, isolate, and do fewer rewarding activities. When sad, mad, or afraid, we generally take worse care of ourselves. Are you noticing a pattern?

Persistent negative emotions also have more direct biological consequences because they can generate toxic stress, and we learned about the dire physiological effects of that in Chapter 3. So not only are negative emotions likely to make everything worse—including pain, ability to function, need for medication, and quality of life—but persistent negative emotions such as depression and anxiety also increase your risk for conditions including heart disease and high blood pressure. Still, having some negative emotions is normal and can be managed. More good news: Positive emotions can buffer the effects of negative emotions. This next part is tricky. Positive emotions can be evasive for many people with chronic pain unless they purposefully train to reset their brains. It's a bit of a harrowing tale. Let's start with what we know about how the brain processes negative emotions and how that processing relates to pain.

Neural Circuitry

The brain processes pain and negative emotions using both shared and independent neural circuitry. When we think of the role of emotions in chronic pain, it's easy to blame depression and anxiety for brain-related changes that promote pain. Yet Felix Brandl and his colleagues at the Technical University of Munich have made such distinctions very clear.[24] They conducted a meta-analysis, a powerful type of study that gathers all possible studies about a related topic and analyzes the data from each separate study as if it were one gigantic study. They identified 320 neuroimaging studies that explored one of three conditions: depression, anxiety, or chronic pain. The team found commonalities in brain processing patterns in all three conditions, but more importantly, they also found distinct differences among the conditions. In chronic pain, a unique neural signature included *fewer* connections between two key brain networks and unique structural changes in the medial temporal lobes, which are key structures for processing memory and pain severity. These findings offer some of the strongest proof to date that pain involves unique brain activity different from depression and anxiety. Once again, your chronic pain isn't simply due to psychiatric illness.

Threats Are Primal and Powerful

While depression and anxiety are distinct processes from chronic pain, some shared brain circuitry helps explain why negative emotions can make your pain worse. As we discussed in the chapter about stress, when something feels threatening, our brains trigger an intense, disorganized, unthinking, primitive response to fight, flight, or freeze. We startle. For survival, all creatures have this startle response. (For some amusing examples, search for "startled cats" on YouTube.)

Imagine walking down an unfamiliar city street at night, alone, feeling uncomfortable. Lurking shadows resemble people or creatures that could harm you. Your heart beats fast, and then somebody taps you on the shoulder. What happens next? Well, you probably look a lot like those startled cats! You nearly jump out of your shoes and scream. Your mind might go blank for a second, your heart races, and you turn to identify the threat so you can fight or run away. You are primed to contend with a threat. Once you discover that it's only a friend saying hello, you sigh with relief, and your parasympathetic nervous system begins to calm your threat-detection system back to normal, although you might still yell at your friend for sneaking up on you in the dark.

The amygdala, a little almond-shaped structure in the brain, drives this fight-flight-or-freeze response. The emotional flooding that occurs when encountering a perceived threat has critical survival value, but it's thoroughly unhelpful when cued by false alarms, such as a critical comment, a mistake at work, or arguing with your significant other. Daniel Goleman refers to this emotional flooding reaction to everyday occurrences or setbacks as amygdala hijack.[25] When we fail to regulate our threatening thoughts and negative emotions, our brains and bodies can process daily stressors as life-threatening events and trigger that biological alarm. Threats are primal, powerful, and not great for your pain. As we know, chronic stress has psychological and physiological consequences, including making your pain worse.

Name, Connect, Reset

Some events in our lives result in thoughts and feelings that seem overwhelming or unacceptable. (*"I shouldn't think or feel that!"*). The next generation of CBT pain therapies include becoming more aware of painful experiences and related emotions, understanding them, and then expressing more adaptive thoughts and feelings so that these brain processes don't amplify or create pain. What do I mean by this? Here's an example that hits close to home.

My husband, Will, is the peanut butter to my jelly, the Yin to my Yang. You get the picture. Out of the blue, my typically healthy, fit, and happy husband developed crippling back pain. We suddenly found ourselves on the other side of the exam room. Now *we* had a chronic pain problem. The pain started in his lower back and radiated down his right leg. The severity forced him to stop whatever he was doing and sit down to catch his breath. Our primary care physician couldn't find an explanation for his pain. The results of a physical exam and MRIs all looked normal. Still, when the pain struck, it was devastating. He'd have days with little or no pain, followed by days with sudden and extreme flares that lasted minutes or hours.

This strange new problem arose while I was a psychology intern in training at Robert Wood Johnson Medical School. I described my husband's pain to my psychology supervisor, Marian Stuart, and she smiled supportively, nodding knowingly. She asked whether I thought that both of Will's parents having terminal cancer might have something to do with it. I didn't see an obvious connection, but—well—maybe? Will adored his parents, as did I, and the day-to-day dreadfulness definitely was taking a toll on his sleep and energy. She instructed me to ask him, the next time he had a flare, what exactly was going through his mind right before the pain began.

It didn't take long for Will to have another episode. He almost collapsed at a shopping mall and gingerly made his way to a bench. Sitting beside him with my hand in his, I asked him what he was thinking about right before the pain began.

He looked confused. "Mom and her cancer."

With a bit of coaxing, he revealed his anger at the disease but also at her for being so stubborn and weak, not her usual strong, feisty, confident self. He was furious and fearful, and he told me that he shouldn't be feeling any of this. He was filled with shame. How could he be mad at her? Then, to our surprise, the moment he named and connected these difficult emotions to his thoughts, the pain subsided and stopped (reset). He acknowledged the painful event, explored unacceptable thoughts, dialed down feelings of threat and fear coming from both the pain and concern about his mom, and allowed himself to experience and then release the difficult emotions.

Of course, the pain came back again throughout the course of his parents' illnesses and many times during the years since, but once he voiced the unacceptable thoughts and emotions and connected the circumstances, the pain reliably stopped. Does this mean that Will made up the pain and it wasn't real? Absolutely not. It was just one of many ways the brain generates pain *on its own*. Some reasonable theories based on neuroscience explain what happens in the brain to make pain like this happen, but we really don't know for sure. Does this mean that something similar might be happening for you? Maybe. Roughly 20 to 30 percent of people with chronic pain might have this type of brain-generated pain, but top-down pain has many manifestations. This is just one of them.

Emotion-Focused CBT

In the 1880s, William James, the father of American psychology, observed that "We often experience emotions not just in our minds but in our bodies as well—in fact, these bodily sensations may be an essential component of an emotional experience." Newer, emotion-focused approaches to chronic pain, such as pain reprocessing therapy (PRT) and emotional awareness and expression therapy (EAET) seem to be helpful for just about everyone with chronic pain, but they can prove particularly effective for people who have pain triggered by negative emotions and thoughts. Both PRT and EAET share therapeutic elements and align with many aspects of the approach in this book. Emotion-focused CBT for pain has four main aspects.

- Understand how the brain amplifies pain and can generate pain completely on its own. That's why we've spent so much time on the neuroscience of pain.
- Know the role that thoughts and emotions play in dialing pain signals up and down. You have the power to change your thoughts and emotions, which means you have the power to influence how your brain processes pain.
- Learn how to name, connect, and reset. Build skills to identify (name) stressful thoughts and feelings, draw associations (connect) among your experience of pain and related thoughts and emotions, and deactivate the false alarm (reset) to help your body and brain regain balance.
- Practice techniques to promote positive emotions, actions, and relationships, the cornerstones of resiliency. As such, think of positive emotions like good medicine.

For your Thriving Plan, you'll learn life skills to help you understand and accept an emotion and then regulate it so that the emotion doesn't regulate you.

The Benefits of Positive Emotions

Positive emotions include forms of happiness—joy, excitement, surprise, delight, cheerfulness—as well as peacefulness: calm, gratitude, confidence, relaxation, and love. These positive emotions play an important part in the pain story, too. Studies exploring positive emotions and pain, where I concentrate much of my research, have shown that joy, laughter, purpose, and social connection effectively buffer the effects of negative emotions and decrease the experience of pain in the brain. People with chronic pain who also have high levels of positive emotion function better and tend to experience less pain. Further, they tend to sleep better, have fewer mental health problems, and lead more fulfilling lives.[26] Why would this be the case?

The "broaden and build" theory of positive emotions might help explain why.[27] When renowned psychologist Barbara Fredrickson was a professor at the University of Michigan, she was one of the first to help us understand that the power of positive emotions might lie in their ability to broaden our repertoires of thought and behavior. When we experience negative emotions, our attention, vision, and thoughts become highly focused. We narrow our options and potential responses. This intense focus has important survival value that helps us spot danger and mount a defense. In contrast, when we feel positive emotions, our field of vision, thought processes, and attention broaden, making us more open, flexible, and creative. Positive emotions also draw people in, which helps us build critical social resources. Under the influence of positive emotions, we are more likely to take good care of ourselves, including eating healthier food, exercising, doing enjoyable activities, building social relationships, and sleeping well. Bottom line: Positive emotions can be good for your mental and physical health.

Positive Emotions Soothe Pain

Your brain has direct connections to your endocrine system, which regulates hormones. When you feel happy, exhilarated, or content, chemicals are released and flow through your body—hooray![28] When you feel happy and excited, several brain structures activate and chit-chat with each other like friends at a party. Collectively these brain areas form the reward processing system. So if you have a positive social experience, win a game, or see something beautiful, your brain registers it as a reward and releases dopamine, for example. Imagine all the partygoers laughing at a funny story at the same time. Reward processing and dopamine release help explain why you might feel sparkly with joy, pride, or excitement when you perceive an object or event as fantastic.

Other happiness messengers include the neurotransmitter serotonin and the hormones oxytocin and endorphins. You likely have heard of serotonin because it is so critical to mood and pain-signal transmission. People with depression, anxiety, trauma, and chronic pain tend to have low levels of serotonin. Oxytocin, the bonding hormone, circulates through our bodies when we feel loving and loved. Endorphins are the body's naturally occurring opioids. When endorphins are released, you feel joyful and maybe a bit giddy, as with a runner's "high." Endorphins cause that high feeling to counter the bodily stress of running. Endorphins are released in other ways, too. Can you recall a time that you laughed so hard that your eyes watered, and you couldn't catch your breath? Afterward, you probably felt tingly or intoxicated, right? Hooray for your body's own, 100 percent natural opioid system! I'd like to prescribe more breathless laughter for you. Here's the kicker. All four of these happiness messengers naturally decrease the experience of pain, *like a drug.*

A Caveat about Positive Emotion and Chronic Pain

Numerous studies have shown that people with chronic pain, depression, anxiety, trauma, and substance addiction can have problems with the reward-processing system in the brain. These problems can result in decreased ability even to recognize positive events as positive. Think of a party where none of the guests chat or even notice one another. That's a lousy party. These same problems with reward-processing circuitry in the brain also impact motivation and result in less active seeking of positive experiences. If you have chronic pain, that phenomenon can help explain that languishing or "meh" feeling even when something good happens.

Take heart, though, because good evidence shows that reward processing can improve through mindfulness, aerobic exercise, connecting with others, savoring the good things in life, gratitude, and intentionally doing enjoyable activities.[29] Part of your chronic pain reset will center on boosting positive emotions by improving how you detect, experience, and seek rewarding events, experiences, and people.

IDEAS TO REMEMBER

- The brain processes emotions and pain with shared and independent circuitry, which is why negative emotions make pain worse and positive emotions can buffer the experience of pain.
- When we fail to regulate threatening thoughts and negative emotions, our brains and bodies see them as life-threatening and trigger false alarms in our stress-response system.
- Name stressful thoughts and feelings. Connect events, thoughts, emotions, and pain. Deactivate false alarms and regain balance.
- Triggered by positive emotions, your body's happiness messengers (dopamine, endorphins, oxytocin, and serotonin) naturally decrease pain.
- Many people with chronic pain have impaired reward-processing circuitry in the brain, but that programming can be reset with positive experiences. So go have some fun!
- A meta-analysis is a powerful study that analyzes data from many different studies about the same topic as if all the data came from one gigantic study.

Lived Experience: Christin

I never saw it coming—then a millisecond of steel, chrome, glass, and excruciating pain. When I was 15, a car hit me while I was riding my bike home from basketball camp. I sustained major injuries, and doctors told my family that it was unlikely that I would survive the night. Thankfully, they were wrong.

Over the next few days, I underwent multiple surgeries, and I spent a month in the hospital. Strenuous physical therapy and additional surgeries over the following year restored my physical function nearly to normal. I'm beyond fortunate not only to be alive but also to be able to talk, walk, and engage in "normal" activities. But my life has never been the same. On the one hand, I gained a new perspective, a sense of purpose, and an appreciation for the gift of life that most people may never understand. On the other hand, my body, mind, and soul experienced severe trauma, leaving me with a new daily companion: chronic pain. Thirty years later, that cruel companion remains.

Due to insufficient awareness of and research on chronic pain, I, like millions of others, have struggled to find knowledgeable healthcare professionals as well as safe and effective treatments. I spent almost a decade experimenting with different drug and nondrug pain treatments to find a combination that helps reduce the severity of my pain without intolerable side effects. The day-to-day grind of trying to function when I look "fine" on the outside but feel constant pain on the inside has taken a toll not just on me but on those with whom I'm closest. The profound impact of my adolescent health experiences prompted me to obtain a science degree and, for the last twenty-five years, to work in the not-for-profit sector as a pain research advocate, but my story doesn't end there.

During a particularly difficult and dark period in my journey, a camera, of all things, changed my life. Now a camera has become my second daily companion. At a time when I didn't have much hope for a meaningful future without significant anguish, I started exploring my surroundings, camera in hand. My love of the ocean drew me to nearby locations that distracted me from physical suffering and began to heal my emotional suffering, while restoring my hope for the future.

I'm drawn to compositions that mimic my life experiences, images that communicate resilience and perseverance despite adversity: rusty, banged-up boats with inspirational names such as *Determination* and *Tenacity*; sturdy lighthouses that have guided people ashore for centuries; unmovable jetties that have withstood the battering of stormy seas; and coastal sunrises that give hope to the weariest of souls. Photography has become a saving grace for me, and I hope that my images encourage others facing any type of adversity that they are stronger than they know and that there's hope for their future—no matter how hopeless the present may feel.

———

Christin Veasley is cofounder and director of the Chronic Pain Research Alliance. Learn more at ChronicPainResearch.org and see her photography at ResiliencePhotography.com.

6

TRAUMA, PAIN, AND HEALING

Bad things happen. A fair amount of adversity occurs in everyone's life. Some adverse events can feel frustrating and stressful, such as missing a plane, while others are more difficult and consequential, such as losing your job. Exceptionally bad events could include a devastating car accident, being the victim of a violent crime, the unexpected death of a loved one, or physical, sexual, or emotional abuse. Trauma is a common reaction to these events and others in which your life feels in peril. Yet psychology and neuroscience tell us that your biology, history, thought patterns, and even the people around you greatly influence your reaction to almost any adverse event and how those reactions might impact you emotionally and physiologically.

Take a moment to review your life. You probably can list at least three perfectly *awful* events that have taken place. Consider writing them down. If you do, rank them from bad to worst or place them in the life stage when they occurred. In other words, did the event take place in childhood, adolescence, or adulthood? Like a scientist, without passion or emotion, recall from the safety of the present the moment you experienced one of these events. Perhaps it completely overwhelmed you, time stood still, you slipped into denial, or you bargained with a higher power. No matter your response, the event became a permanent part of your life story. Maybe some of these traumatic events caused you great distress that disrupted your life. You might have suffered terribly and wondered whether you ever could get to the other side.

OK, now step away from this thought experiment and note how you feel. Even though the event may have taken place a long time ago and you tried to remain emotionally distanced, you likely still felt something perhaps quite strong, such as intense fear. The emotions tied to these events survive for years and even decades. Your brain often encodes threatening events in your memory with exceptional precision so that you avoid similar situations and survive in the future. Gee, thanks, brain.

Trauma leaves unique marks on brain and body. Even changes at the DNA level can take place when you experience extreme and persistent adversity, loss, fear, and trauma. As we saw in the stress chapter, the body pays a heavy price for the persistent activation of the stress-response system.

Take a deep, slow breath and release those events as you exhale. Seriously, inhale deeply and, when you breathe out, let the memories go. Imagine them going into a box placed on a hidden shelf. Now let's talk.

Adversity and Trauma

Many people with chronic pain report that a traumatic event, such as a car accident, emergency surgery, or a terrible loss preceded their pain. Others may have endured childhood abuse, neglect, or social alienation and, because trauma begets trauma, many experience abuse and other forms of trauma in adulthood as well. This stressful environment sets in motion slow-boiling physiological changes that can form the biological foundation for the development of chronic pain.

Studies have shown that trauma experienced during childhood or adulthood correlates with increased physical sensitivity to painful stimuli.[30] In other words, the brain more readily screams, *"Pain!"* The good news is that the same biological systems that changed in response to those stressful events are, for the most part, malleable like clay and thus subject to changing again. Our ever-advancing understanding of the brain and its remarkable plasticity informs new treatments and hope that many different approaches can decrease pain and improve well-being. You—yes, you—can foster these changes by what you do going forward.

We humans are remarkably resilient. Research exploring our ability to bounce back after traumatic events is compelling. Initially, we might feel stunned and lost but, more often than not, we find a way to lean on our resources and find our emotional footing once again, thus restoring balance. As we have discussed already, how well we rebound from setbacks depends on reliable social support and healthy coping skills. If these resilience resources are minimal or dysfunctional (unsupportive family or friends, substance use, denial), we are more likely to experience trauma and toxic stress.

Before we focus on how resilient people cope with adversity, I want to make sure you're safe. Some types of adversity are tougher to weather than others and can result in a trauma reaction. If you've experienced traumatic events and never sought support or have symptoms of post-traumatic stress disorder (PTSD), this book could help, but there are more effective treatments for your recovery. See the Resources section on page 255, and I encourage you to use the phone numbers and websites there to help you find a therapist in your area who can support you better than I can here.

Maintaining Perspective

Nothing can change the fact that traumatic events have happened in your life. In the 1979 film *Superman*, Clark Kent discovers that his love, Lois Lane, has died. Distraught, he cradles her in his arms, holding her limp body close to his chest, and, as Superman, he flies counterclockwise around the Earth. With increasing speed, he circles the planet in a blur until he halts and then reverses time. This desperate act allows him to travel through time to relive the moments before her death to stop it from happening. The desire to reverse time and stop bad events from happening is universal, which makes this an iconic moment in film. But none of us is

Superman, so we must find a way to cope with adversity, loss, trauma, and failure and, if we really want to thrive, perhaps even grow from it.

An important aspect of recovery from difficult life events is thinking about them differently over time. Trauma can change the way you view the world, often in profound ways, but thoughts evolve over time as you integrate new information and experiences into your understanding of your life. As your thoughts evolve, your emotional reactions tend to change, too. For example, when people lose their jobs, they initially may think, *This is awful! I'm such a loser. Who will ever hire me again?* Angry, despondent thoughts are the go-to reaction for many people; catastrophizing, self-denigration, and feeling numb are common. But with support from friends and a clear head for reflection, we might come to the realization that those initial thoughts weren't true. When that happens, our emotional state improves as well. We then find ourselves in a better position to search for a new job and perhaps even find one that pays better and where we feel more appreciated and fulfilled. In the heat of catastrophe mode, though, the possibility that the loss might result in a better situation seems like sheer madness.

No matter the event, research tells us that the traumatic event itself matters less to our health than the psychological distress that we experience after the event. The level of distress determines whether your brain and body will experience the event as tolerable or toxic stress.

Find Your Way Back

Even in the face of adversity, a road to happiness still exists. Deep in loss and despair, it's hard to believe that you won't always feel terrible, but it's almost always true. The worst of the fear can pass, but this may require hard work and good care provided by trained mental healthcare providers. Most of the painful feelings of loss can pass, too, after we take the time to grieve the loss and care for ourselves. It's also critical to practice self-compassion and seek social and even professional help when needed. Again, check out the Resources section of this book for possibilities.

After accepting and processing terrible events, people sometimes even experience post-traumatic *growth*. Such post-traumatic growth happens with people, say, who survive a life-threatening illness or accident and feel that they now have a gift, an opportunity to lead lives that feel more meaningful and rewarding than before. Think about Christin who we met before this chapter and her recovery from being hit by a car. We also see this in the case of parents who lose a child and find purpose and even strength through becoming advocates to decrease the likelihood that other children or parents will suffer in a similar way. Such people bravely find ways to face their fear, mourn, and then grow in the shadow of disaster. Studies have shown that the people most likely to experience post-traumatic growth are those with strong social support, healthy coping strategies, and good mental and physical health.[31] This book helps you build these critical skills and resources.

Embrace Your Scars and Imperfections

Leonard Cohen sings that the cracks in things are valuable because they allow in the light. Trauma can change you forever in countless ways. Perhaps now you can view some of the most negative events in your life and see how you have grown from them emotionally or spiritually. Inspired by what you learned through adversity, you might even behave differently now. Our scars, hidden or visible, make us unique. A Japanese aesthetic called wabi-sabi finds beauty inherent in asymmetry, rough edges, unfinished work, and even broken or mended objects. In nature, such objects are intriguing, relatable, and beautiful. The same worldview holds true for us humans. Your imperfections make you intriguing, relatable, and beautiful. Embrace your scars and imperfections. Revel in being a work in progress. You don't need to be perfect to be exquisite and loved.

Appreciate Your Failures and Maintain a Growth Mindset

No discussion of adversity can avoid mentioning failure, which represents a very personal form of adversity. Some failures can be devastating, but failure doesn't mean that you're inadequate or incompetent. No one gets through life without a few spectacular mistakes and blunders. What matters is how you think about these unfortunate events and what you do going forward. Will you worry about them obsessively, replay them endlessly in your head, cursing your stupidity? Or will you reflect, maybe blush or laugh, permit yourself a little self-compassion, and learn from your failure? The latter approach avoids a lot of unproductive thoughts and negative feelings and can help ensure success the next time around. Oh yeah, you'll also sleep better, feel happier, and experience less pain.

Carol Dweck discusses our reactions to failure in the terms of having a growth mindset (or not).[32] She proposes that some people believe that ability and potential are fixed. Either you're talented or not. In contrast, others have a growth mindset, in which they believe that they can develop ability and talent through hard work. People with a fixed mindset take failure hard because it means that they've reached the limit of their abilities, whereas people with a growth mindset use failure as feedback. If they fail, they might use this observation to keep pushing toward success. I encourage you to cultivate a growth mindset, especially when you try the activities in Part Two.

Grieve the Losses but Surround Yourself with Nourishing People and Activities

Feedback from those around you heavily determines how you envision your failures, how you feel about your prospects, and how you think about yourself. Surrounding yourself with individuals who believe in you, support you, and encourage you to succeed is *critical* to your health and happiness. We'll explore social connectedness in greater depth shortly.

How you react to adversity largely determines whether you'll suffer or thrive. Now, that's not to say that you simply can think happy thoughts and the difficulty will go away. That would be awesome, but it doesn't work that way. You need to experience the event to the best of your ability. Feel the hurt, anger, frustration, or loss and put honest words to those emotions. Then, ugh, the hard part: Find a way to accept that the event happened. Grieve. That grief might last a few minutes or a few years. For overwhelming or persistent grief, seek support and guidance from a mental healthcare professional, but for more manageable losses, ask for help from family and friends to find the other side. Either way, the key is to make sense of the event using your incredible ability to think.

IDEAS TO REMEMBER

- Enduring adversity is an unavoidable part of the human experience.
- How you think about an event matters more than the event itself.
- A history of trauma is common in people with chronic pain and impacts the experience of pain at biological, psychological, emotional, and behavioral levels.
- An important aspect of recovery from traumatic events is thinking about them differently over time; finding a new sense of purpose can be one of the best outcomes.
- Embrace your failures and imperfections. They make you wiser, more relatable, more lovable, and definitely more interesting.

Lived Experience: Kevin

"Tense the muscles in your jaw, hold, and then release," said the clinical psychologist, guiding me to tense and relax all the muscles in my body, from head to toe. Afterward, I felt calmer, clearer, and more at ease. I wanted to learn more and started listening to guided meditations on mindfulness and progressive muscle relaxation. After a few months, I was delighted to realize that I had found valuable tools for managing my fibromyalgia symptoms.

Six years earlier, Dr. Dan Clauw, who you already met in this book, diagnosed me with fibromyalgia. This diagnosis followed thirteen dreadful months of fear and agonizing worry over inexplicably worsening and spreading pain and sleep problems—all of which made me feel like my body was under siege by an invisible, insidious force. As a twenty-one-year-old man, I had envisioned finishing college with a diploma, not a chronic pain diagnosis. But with Dan's guidance, I learned more about fibromyalgia and developed tools to manage my symptoms. These included medications, such as cyclobenzaprine and medical cannabis, and lifestyle strategies, including eating more plant-based foods, yoga, massage, and establishing a consistent sleep schedule. Improvement felt slow, but these tools worked wonders over time. My body grew stronger. I finished college, landed a full-time job, bought a house, and got married.

Despite this wonderful growth, my relationship with pain remained fraught. I thought that fibromyalgia pain was maladaptive, served no purpose, and should be avoided. Consequently, pain and fear of pain jealously hoarded my attention, and I relentlessly chastised myself for any decisions that worsened my symptoms.

Life continued, and I started a doctoral program in public health. Midway through my program, I pulled a muscle during a game of kickball, initiating a year-long pain flare. I was miserable. My previous tools weren't working. I got massages, went to physical therapy, and saw a dietician. After tracking my diet, stress levels, and pain symptoms, I was struck by the close relationship between stress and pain. The data don't lie, and I finally saw that my thoughts profoundly influenced my pain. It wasn't enough to work only with my physical body; I needed to work with my mind. I sought the help of a clinical psychologist.

Our sessions provided perspective on my internal monologue around my symptoms: how it worsened physical pain through unconscious physiological reactions (tensing muscles, breathing shallowly) and how my laser focus on pain often enforced a dichotomy on bodily sensations, namely: painful versus not painful. Inspired by these insights and wanting to go deeper, I trained to become a yoga teacher during my final year of graduate school.

In addition to learning yoga practices and philosophy, I worked with my teacher to connect those practices to my own understanding of pain and fibromyalgia. One key takeaway was the importance of taking a pause—no matter how small—before reacting. When encountering something unfamiliar or scary, my mind often jumped to *"Pain! Bad! Stop!"* and I withdrew. Pausing summoned space and courage, allowing me to practice bypassing the artificial pain dichotomy and to explore edgy feelings that typically landed in the "pain" category: physical or emotional discomfort, agitation, and unease. To my surprise, I found that the borders between pain and discomfort are flexible not fixed. Through my training and experience, I deliberately practiced becoming more skillful at discerning the difference.

Through these evolving practices, I have been reframing my understanding of fibromyalgia. I've come to see fibromyalgia as a trait of heightened sensitivity rather than a painful, inexplicable burden or a diagnosis that needs fixing. This sensitivity is integral to my life and my being. It's not an enemy but part of me—one that I am learning to love more with each passing day.

Kevin Boehnke is a research assistant professor in the Chronic Pain and Fatigue Research Center in the Department of Anesthesiology at the University of Michigan.

7

MINDFULNESS AND THE
POWER OF PRESENCE

As we have learned, persistent, toxic stress is a detriment to your happiness and health. It can create or worsen anxiety, muscle tension, insomnia, irritability, racing thoughts, sadness, fatigue, headaches, lack of motivation, and upset stomach. Stress creates the perfect bodily environment for your pain to fester and grow. So I hope you'll consider addressing the stress in your life as a priority.

We can decrease our stress in many ways, and you'll try a lot of them in the second part of this book. One of the most studied approaches is mindfulness-based stress reduction (MBSR). Often offered at academic medical centers, MBSR teaches people how to practice mindfulness meditation in class and at home. Studies have shown MBSR to be effective for decreasing stress and chronic pain as well as helpful for improving functioning and quality of life in a wide range of diseases and conditions such as heart disease, high blood pressure, cancer, asthma, sleep disturbances, skin problems, stomach conditions, fatigue, anxiety, depression, thick toenails, and hairy eyeballs. OK, I made up the last two to see if you were paying attention and to underline the point that mindfulness can be helpful for just about everything.

Still, it's not a substitute for regular medical care. But when added to an existing treatment program, it can improve quality of life. Mindfulness practices can involve a weeks-long, in-person program, but you can benefit from a less formal practice such as listening to guided imagery recordings or regularly practicing mindful breathing. In whatever form, mindfulness practices center on teaching you how to be more present.

What Does It Mean to Be Present?

Have you ever noticed someone suddenly tune out in the middle of a conversation? The person might be looking right at you, but his eyes aren't really connecting with yours. Perhaps the person is trying to recall a similar discussion or helpful information that pertains to your story, but it's equally possible that he just remembered that he needs to buy bananas.

Human minds merrily flit from one thought to the next, from the past to present, from the future to bananas. Yogis and yoginis, the kings and queens of meditation, refer to this distracted state as having "monkey mind." The term vividly describes how the mind jumps from one thought to another like a monkey jumping from one tree branch to another to another *to another*. When your mind exists in this frenetic state, it's impossible to stay focused or exist in the present moment. It's difficult to counter distracting thoughts that pop up and demand attention like a bright shiny obj—*Oooooo, what's that?*

Mindfulness refers to the ability to stay grounded in the present, fully aware of where you are, with whom you're talking, and what you're doing and feeling right *now*. When mindful, you aren't overreacting to or feeling overwhelmed by what's happening around you. It just is. Jon Kabat-Zinn, a professor emeritus at the University of Massachusetts Medical School and commonly credited as the creator of MBSR, defines mindfulness as "awareness that arises through paying attention, on purpose, in the present moment, nonjudgmentally." Our tendency—as thinking, self-referential humans—to take ourselves too darn seriously typically explains this lack of ability to be calm, focused, and present. This state of mind can result in constantly searching for threats and detecting threats that don't exist anywhere but in our minds. As we've learned, stressful thoughts have bodily consequences that worsen pain, among other physical and psychological harms.

Mindfulness for People with Pain

MBSR stands on the premise that it's possible to live in the moment and become fully aware of your inner world and outer experiences. You learn how to observe your thoughts, feelings, and bodily experiences from a distance, like a scientist, without judging them. Like pain, they merely are happening in that moment. (*"Hmmm, interesting."*) Such nonjudgmental awareness in daily life helps promote serenity and clarity and can help you experience more joy. When calm and centered, you are better able to access your inner resiliency resources that can help you solve problems, manage stress, and even heal more effectively.

For chronic pain, MBSR helps bring your attention to the present, even when what's happening in the present is the sensory experience of pain. You can consider pain from a distance, too. Picture yourself as an emotionally neutral scientist or Vulcan observing that pain is happening in this moment. (*"Fascinating."*) When you exist in a single moment in time, you may have a more nuanced understanding of what's taking place in your body. In any given moment, the brain is processing millions of pieces of input beyond your pain, such as sounds in the environment, visual stimuli, scents, air temperature, the feel of your clothes and shoes, and about ten possible itch locations across your body. Take a second right now and think about where you might itch. I bet that at least one place came immediately to mind— maybe more. The brain uses the process of attention to screen out all but the most salient sensory experiences, which is a critical function. Taking in everything all the time would feel completely overwhelming!

Still, with all that information coming into your brain in a given moment, why does it feel like you can experience only pain? Well, pain is a narcissist and screams for your attention like a spoiled child. It serves a critical survival function, and by nature your brain pays attention to it to ensure your survival. But chronic pain represents good wiring gone bad. So what do you do? Acknowledge the spoiled child without judgment and then heed other, more "deserving" children, such as the sound of the wind in the trees, the color of the sky, your pet's fuzzy ears, or the delicious taste of a piece of fresh fruit. You already have the power to choose what you notice, and really you can attend to only one thing at a time. It just takes a bit of practice to send pain signals into the background.

With mindfulness, you also can become more aware of unhelpful negative thoughts and emotions that accompany your pain. Separate fear avoidance and worst-case scenarios from the chatter and take them to task. Let mindfulness help you identify and differentiate pain from the negativity that mixes with sensory signals to make the pain feel more severe, distressing, and disabling. Mindfulness also can help you take a broader perspective, focusing less on the pain and more on neutral, pleasant, or, as Kevin might put it, "edgy" pain experiences.

Mindfulness Practices

MBSR and similar practices rely on mindfulness meditation, meaning practices to focus your attention in the present. Activities include short or long meditations and body-awareness activities such as a body scan (searching each part of your body for tension and releasing it) and walking meditation. All activities teach you how to exist more in the moment, nonjudgmentally aware of your body, thoughts, and feelings, to help you better understand and change your experience of pain. MBSR also includes gentle stretching exercises similar to tai chi or qigong. These movements increase mindful awareness of your body. (They're not geared toward building strength, flexibility, or fitness.) Breathing also plays a central role in mindfulness practices. Here, too, slowing down, turning inward, and experiencing breathing in a pleasant way can enhance your sense of being present.

Too often we scarf our meals, not recognizing how much we're consuming, how good (or bad) the food tastes, or its benefits for body and mind. Mindful eating, frequently a part of MBSR, teaches you how to slow down when eating and to use all five senses to appreciate your food. Savoring food provides an opportunity to enjoy the experience and often results in eating less. You'll have the opportunity to try mindful eating in the second part of this book. I think you'll like it.

The Benefits of Mindfulness

Numerous studies support mindfulness practices for chronic pain, commonly finding improvement in pain, depression, and health-related quality of life. In a landmark study published in the *Journal of the American Medical Association*, a team led by Daniel Cherkin at the University of Washington in Seattle found that people with chronic low back pain who were assigned randomly to take an eight-session MBSR program had greater reductions in disability compared to people who received standard care for their pain.[33] The study also found that people in the MBSR group rated their pain as less bothersome than those in the control group. Most encouragingly, the researchers observed that the benefits of MBSR were still present a year later!

Many more studies show the benefits for people with pain, including an encouraging one conducted by researchers at Duke University and the University of North Carolina. These investigators explored the effectiveness of MBSR for modifying pain and psychological symptoms in women with a history of abuse early in life.[34] People who have experienced early-life trauma have an increased risk for stress-response system dysfunction, increased sensitivity to pain, and a sharply elevated risk for depression, anxiety, and other mental health problems. The research team noted MBSR-related improvements in participants' pain sensitivity as well as improved mindfulness and emotion regulation. Would you take a pill that resulted in less pain, better functioning, and decreased emotional distress and lasted a *year*? I bet you would, but name one pill that does that. There isn't one.

OK, But How Does Mindfulness Help?

The amazing human capacity to time-travel mentally—thinking about the past or the future—can aid learning, put information into context, and enable planning. It often happens automatically, and decades of research have shown that mental time travel isn't always beneficial. Sometimes it can add a lot of stress to our lives. Research shows that thoughts too focused on the past tend to result in depression, while thoughts too focused on the future tend to promote anxiety.

Amplify either thought pattern with rumination, and you have a truly harmful situation. We don't yet understand completely how mindfulness practices help relieve pain and improve mood and functionality, but it seems that just having better awareness of our thoughts and recognizing that these thoughts are transient mental events can be helpful. In other words, our lives tend to improve when we recognize that not all thoughts are true—many of them more pessimistic than necessary—and simply choose to ignore them. You might notice that, if you ignore them, they tend to fade away. This new perspective meaningfully can decrease thought processes such as pain catastrophizing and rumination. Remember, with fewer negative thoughts come fewer negative emotions. Without all that negativity, your mind-space has a wee bit of room for more positive thoughts (*"Maybe I can decrease my pain."*) and feelings of calm, joy, and hope.

Mindfulness practices also correlate with changes in the brain. You might think that brain activity would register low in the meditating mind, but we see many areas of the brain light up as if in a state of engagement and readiness. In a meta-analysis, Maddalena Boccia and her colleagues at Sapienza University of Rome extracted data from more than 100 studies.[35] They found that meditation activates brain areas involved in self-regulation, problem-solving, adaptive behavior, and interoception (awareness of internal bodily processes). Their analysis also reported that, selecting only for expert meditators, meditation practice had an association with functional and structural brain changes in areas involved in self-regulation and self-awareness. In another scientific paper, Fadel Zeidan and his colleagues reported that, after as few as ten hours of practice, mindfulness-based pain relief correlated with higher-order changes in the brain.[36] These changes took place in brain areas associated with reappraisal, which is the process of reconsidering the meaning of something in a more positive light.

What If Meditation Isn't for You?

Good question, glad you asked! If meditation isn't your thing, you still can learn how to be more present. In our studies, we've encountered people who voice concerns about meditation from a religious perspective. Meditation, a practice that goes back thousands of years, forms part of many religions, including Hinduism, Buddhism, Judaism, and Christianity. Some who pray can adapt prayer in a way to allow them to be still, in the moment, and become aware of bodily experiences, feelings, and thoughts before or after they pray.

Meditation itself makes others feel anxious. This common phenomenon can occur even among seasoned meditators and makes a lot of sense. Mindfulness practice isn't about putting on rose-colored glasses or hanging out in your happy place. It's about being fully present with your feelings, emotions, and thoughts. A study led by Jarad Lindahl at Brown University explored potentially negative effects associated with meditation.[37] Investigators conducted in-depth interviews with sixty regular practitioners of meditation and found that some experienced transient feelings of fear, anxiety, panic, or paranoia when meditating or soon after practice. These emotions starkly oppose the calm, peacefulness, clarity, and comfort most people report when meditating and can make practice frustrating or unhelpful. If you gave meditation a try and it made you feel panicky, anxious, or lousy, you're not alone. Alternatives to meditation can help you achieve a more mindful, pleasant state.

Other Paths to Mindfulness

A key element of meditation is quieting the mind, turning chatter into whispers, and whispers into peace. Many methods can achieve this result. Mindful walking differs from a typical stroll in that you intend to make it part of your wellness practice. For example, you become aware of your breath and the act of walking, feeling your legs moving, muscles tensing and releasing, and your feet touching the ground. Engage all your senses. What do you see, smell, hear, and feel? When thoughts arise, let them float away.

Another mindfulness practice that doesn't involve meditation is guided imagery, which involves listening to recorded descriptions of beautiful, peaceful places or affirmative narratives that promote relaxation and well-being. The simplest way to engage in this practice is to download a free app, such as Insight Timer. Recordings range from one minute to longer than an hour. I recommend recordings of fifteen minutes or fewer in case you fall asleep.

Lastly, you also can engage in a hobby that you love, one that's so engrossing that you lose track of time while doing it, such as playing a musical instrument; painting, coloring, or drawing; assembling a jigsaw puzzle; knitting, quilt making, or other needle crafts; gardening; or even golf. Whatever you love you can make a mindful activity just by recognizing where you are and what you're doing in the moment, moment by moment. Engage all your senses, become aware of your breath and body, and allow your thoughts to pass without judgment or concern. Think about how one or more mindfulness practices might fit into your daily life.

IDEAS TO REMEMBER

- Mindfulness means your ability to stay in the present, fully aware of where you are and what you are doing and with whom. In a mindful state, you don't feel overwhelmed by what's happening around you.
- Mindfulness-Based Stress Reduction (MBSR) is a more formal program that has mindfulness at its core. MBSR has been shown to be helpful for people with chronic pain.
- MBSR brings your attention to the present, even if your primary sensory experience is pain. In MBSR, you consider pain from a distance, with interest and not dread.
- Mindfulness includes more than just meditation. You can pay attention to the present while breathing, walking, singing, dancing, eating, and just about any other activity. All you need to do is exist in the present for a while.

8

SLEEP, YOUR FICKLE FRIEND

I'm a psychology intern at Trenton Psychiatric Hospital in New Jersey. In the old, imposing stone buildings, you almost can hear the whispers of past patients. A locked unit in a more modern building houses only women. On this ward, most of them have a history of violence, from simple assault to grisly murder.

I walk briskly up the hall in jarring white light. The corridor smells like rubbing alcohol and coffee that has sat on a warming burner for too long. I hear a menacing voice behind me.

"Where you goin' in such a hurry?" she asks, closing fast.

This patient has a history of violence, and now I'm imagining the worst. About twenty feet on the left, behind a locked door, lies the safety of a therapy room. Even if another staff member is working with a patient there, I'm ducking into it.

"Hey, intern, come here. I have something for you. Wanna see?"

I could yell, "code grey" or shout for help, but the stench of weakness would cling to me for the rest of my time on the wards. I walk faster.

"Now, you're making me *angry*, little doctor."

My trembling hands are flipping through my keys, five steps to go, and *oh-my-God, oh-my-God,* I can't find the key.

"Having problems with your keys, *innnnnn*-tern?"

Her hand swipes at my hair as the key turns in the lock. On the other side of the door, her ashen face presses against the safety glass. She's laughing, no, *howling,* and—

I'm awake. Monday morning, 3:17 a.m., sweating, thirsty, and terrified, heart pounding. This is the fourth or fifth Sunday that this has happened. For hours, sleep evades me . . . until it doesn't. Then vivid nightmares transport me to that terrifying day. My acute, situational insomnia strikes only on Sunday nights. I always have been a world-class sleeper. Now I'm not, and it *sucks.*

Bad Sleep Is a Nightmare

Acute insomnia affects almost a quarter of Americans each year. For many people, insomnia fortunately resolves on its own once a specific stressor is gone, or it improves with minor behavioral changes. In contrast, chronic insomnia affects around 10 to 15 percent of people and seriously disrupts functioning and well-being. Insomnia and poor sleep, in general, occur regularly in most people with chronic pain. As many as 70 percent of people with chronic pain report some type of sleep disturbance.[38]

Over time, the occurrence and severity of insomnia can wax and wane, but it remains a too-frequent disruptive bedfellow. Some people fall asleep just fine but wake in the wee hours and find themselves unable to fall back to sleep. Many people with chronic pain wake up not feeling refreshed, no matter how many hours of sleep they get. Formal sleep studies comparing people with chronic pain to healthy volunteers affirm these subjective experiences of poor sleep. Sleep apnea and restless legs syndrome also commonly occur in people with chronic pain.[39] Whatever the disturbance, the consequences look the same: daytime sleepiness, fatigue, cognitive fogginess, depression or apathy, and greater pain.

Poor Sleep Worsens Pain

Evidence suggests that sleep deprivation may amplify the perception of existing pain, but new data suggest the effect could be more direct. In a study conducted by Mathew Walker and Adam Krause at the University of California at Berkley, they systematically deprived healthy volunteers of sleep and found that sleep deprivation increased their sensitivity to pain.[40] This change in sensitivity intriguingly resulted in corresponding changes in how the brain processed pain signals. Another key finding: brain areas that help release dopamine and other neurochemicals that promote pain relief showed less activity.

Beyond feeling lousy and being more sensitive to pain, chronic poor sleep appears to pose a threat to your general health and this threat may flow through your immune system. A rich body of evidence connects sleep to changes in immune function. Studies show that a good night's sleep after a dose of vaccine boosts its effectiveness, while poor sleep after vaccination weakens the immune response. Other studies suggest that long-term sleep deprivation increases the risk for diabetes, heart disease, and dementia. Chronic inflammation driven by poor sleep could be the culprit.[41]

Pain, sleep, and depression are three of the SPACE symptoms often present in people with chronic pain. All these symptoms interact with one another, but sleep is the most influential of the trio. Yes, sleep might matter more to your health and well-being than the pain you feel. Indulge me for a moment. Imagine the SPACE symptoms as a dragon, with sleep as the head and the other four symptoms the legs. Now, tell me how you'd defeat the dragon. In your specific case, if sleep is a problem *at all*, you attack that part of the dragon first. But you need to go into battle with the proper weapons. Let's arm ourselves by taking stock of what might be disrupting healthy restorative sleep.

What Keeps You Up at Night?

Many activities contribute to poor sleep, including going to bed and waking up at different times; staying in bed, tossing and turning, when sleep doesn't come; using laptops, mobile devices, or anything that projects blue light right before bedtime; consuming caffeine late in the day; having stressful conversations close to bedtime; sleeping with rambunctious pets; sleeping with restless or snoring bed partners; and so on. A thorough list of tips to address these common sleep-defeating behaviors appears at the end of this chapter.

Your pain itself can make sleep almost impossible at times, whether you can't get comfortable enough to fall asleep or pain wakes you in the middle of the night. Some pain diagnoses relate to changes in problems with your sleep architecture. For example, people with fibromyalgia appear to often have periods of wakefulness during non-REM sleep that might explain why many with fibromyalgia can sleep for seven or eight hours but wake feeling exhausted.

Experiencing pain that makes it hard to doze off can trigger stressful thoughts. Those thoughts lead us to one of the most powerful stimulants keeping you awake at night: your *way*-too-chatty mind. The thoughts you think before you lay your head on the pillow set the stage for how likely you will fall asleep. If your thoughts flow quietly and pleasantly, like a lazy mountain stream, you will have the calm you need to sleep. On the other hand, if your thoughts are rushing like white-water rapids, well, that turbulent state will make sleep almost impossible. So why is that?

Think back to our discussion of cognitive-behavioral therapy. Thoughts come first and trigger emotions that lead to responses or behaviors. In the case of sleep, tortured thoughts raise feelings of fear, regret, anger, and sadness. In this state, the stress-response system activates. Neurochemicals such as adrenaline pump through your body and worsen an already heightened state of being. Now, your body is on full alert, vigilant to whatever threat, human or otherwise, your brain is sure will pounce.

Yes, we are an evolved species, but our brains still have ancient structures and functions better suited for roaming the veldt thousands of years ago. This physiological vulnerability means that we need to use the evolved aspects of our brains to reassure the primitive parts. We'll learn techniques—paced breathing, mindfulness, guided imagery, progressive muscle relaxation, positive reflection, and more—in Part Two to help you calm your busy, primitive brain and improve your pain at the same time.

Turn Off the Light!

Circadian rhythms refer to the body's natural, twenty-four-hour cycles that cue daily functions and processes. The most well-known one is the sleep-wake cycle. When working properly, this circadian rhythm results in reliable, restorative sleep. When this rhythm falls out of sync, you incur greater risks for insomnia, diabetes, obesity, depression, and bipolar disorder. Unfortunately, it's easy to disrupt the biological clock that sets your circadian rhythms. Too little light during the day or too much light at night can ruin your sleep.

A study from the lab of Phyllis Zee, director of the Center for Circadian and Sleep Medicine at Northwestern University, found that allowing even a little light into the room at night resulted in participants having elevated heart rates throughout the night, suggesting low-level stress-response system activation.[42] This light exposure, albeit minor, led to increased insulin resistance the next morning. The sleepers all reported sleeping well, but the light exposure still had adverse physiological effects. Taking all studies in this area together gives us crystal-clear marching orders: get lots of natural light exposure in the morning and sleep in the dark at night.

Take Stock with a Sleep Diary

If you're not a great sleeper, I'm going to ask you to do something for the next seven days. Please keep a sleep diary. It's an easy task. Put paper and a pen or pencil by your bed and, first thing in the morning, before your morning routine begins, make some notes that answer these questions:

- What time did you go to bed, and what time did you wake?
- Did you fall asleep right away?
- If not, how long did you lie in bed awake?
- What kept you awake?
- Did you sleep through the night?

- If not, how often did you wake, and what woke you?
- Were you able to fall back asleep?
- If not, what happened?—for example: pain, worry, clock watching, hunger, TV, smartphone, cat.
- Did you wake feeling refreshed?
- How many hours did you sleep?
- If your sleep didn't feel refreshing, what might have gotten in the way?

Control the Controllable

Sleep is so important that I would like you to start addressing it *now*. Yes, before you begin the program in Part Two. If you *always* wake, feeling refreshed and perky, skip to the next chapter. If you develop sleep problems later, you can come back here. People with sleep apnea, restless leg syndrome, or other serious sleep disorders should seek evaluation and treatment from healthcare providers. For everyone else, here's what you can change right now.

The list below supports healthy sleep. Check anything you already do and think about what you can do to adopt the healthy practices that you didn't check. You have chronic pain, so some of these tips may not suit you perfectly. Feel free to adapt them to accommodate your specific situation. For example, if getting out of bed when you don't fall asleep right away might cause more pain and trouble than it's worth, sit up and scoot to the other side of the bed to read for a bit. Doing that allows you to change your sleep context without triggering more pain.

Sleep-Enhancing Practices

Check all the boxes below that apply to you right now.

- ☐ I make sleep a priority.
- ☐ I wake up around the same time every morning, even on weekends.
- ☐ I go to bed around the same time each night, even on weekends.
- ☐ During the day, I get lots of natural light, especially in the morning.
- ☐ I consume no caffeine (including chocolate!) within ten hours of bedtime.

☐ I limit my alcohol intake and don't drink within a couple hours of bedtime.

☐ I follow a calming nightly routine (put on pajamas, brush teeth, read for thirty minutes, etc.).

☐ I avoid laptop, tablet, and smartphone use at least thirty to sixty minutes before bed.

☐ I wind down thirty minutes before bed by doing something relaxing.

☐ I dim the lights thirty minutes before bedtime to aid my body's production of melatonin.

☐ I go to bed only when feeling sleepy.

☐ My bedroom is quiet, the temperature comfortably cool and pleasant.

☐ When I turn the lights off, my bedroom is dark (no alarm-clock glow).

☐ My bed is comfortable, and my pillows are perfect for me.

☐ I use my bed only for sleep and sex, not for watching TV, paying bills, working, or other activities.

☐ I use sleep techniques such as paced breathing or guided imagery.

☐ I think about things that make me feel grateful or happy right before I close my eyes.

☐ If I don't fall asleep right away, I get back up and do something pleasant but not stimulating; then I go back to bed when I feel sleepy.

☐ My healthcare provider has reviewed the timing of any medications I take, and I take them in ways that will enhance sleep.

To Nap or Not to Nap

That is the question. Who would've thought that napping was controversial? Some experts recommend avoiding naps entirely when trying to stabilize your sleep. Others say a short nap can help. My colleagues, who spend a lot of time thinking about improving sleep in the context of chronic pain, suggest that an occasional nap of no more than twenty minutes is fine. That time limit is firm, so set an alarm and, when it goes off, get up right away. Never use the snooze button, which trains your body to expect interrupted sleep.

The #1 Tip for Improving Sleep

Establish a fixed sleep schedule, also known as *sleep time stabilization*. That's the most effective task you can do right now to improve your sleep. Our brains and bodies love predictability and naturally function on a clock that releases hormones at set intervals to regulate everything from hunger and digestion to wakefulness and agility. Go to bed and get up at the same time *every day*. Yes, that means weekends, too. Varying those sleep times by even an hour won't get the job done. Give it a try for a week or two and see what happens. What have you got to lose?

IDEAS TO REMEMBER

- Most people with chronic pain experience sleep disturbances, and poor sleep makes pain and other symptoms worse. Poor sleep affects how the brain processes pain.
- Sleep is the lowest-hanging fruit of treatment options for chronic pain. If you can sleep well again, your pain, mood, energy, and ability to think clearly likely will improve, too.
- Bad habits undermine good sleep. Changing even just a few of those bad habits can make a *big* difference.
- Go to sleep and wake at the same time every day, even on weekends.

9

EXERCISE IS A WONDER DRUG

The scientific evidence is overwhelming. Thousands of studies demonstrate the remarkable power of exercise to improve physical health, including decreasing your risk for common diseases and conditions such as heart disease, diabetes, cancer, obesity, and of course chronic pain. With better overall health, exercisers tend to outlive non-exercisers. In addition to the physical benefits, studies document psychological and emotional benefits, as well. People who exercise regularly are less likely to feel sad, lonely, depressed, anxious, or stressed. They're happier, healthier, and live longer. Sounds pretty good, right?

If exercise is a wonder drug, why doesn't everyone do it all the time? The healthcare industry struggles with that question constantly! For chronic pain, I want to show you how exercise might help you in particular. Remember, people with top-down pain should engage in activities that impact brain function. Exercise clearly results in impressive brain changes and promotes the release of endorphins that can make you feel joyful and decrease your pain. If you don't exercise regularly already, my job is to help you formulate a plan to get you moving that's accessible, sustainable, and fun for you.

Exercise has more benefits than just physical fitness. Exercise can improve flexibility, range of motion, balance, and strength, all critical for maintaining function and successful aging. Exercise is also good for your brain! During exercise, your muscles release myokines, a kind of messenger protein, into the bloodstream. Recent research shows that myokines may support memory, learning, and mood.[43] We are constantly learning more about how the body and the brain communicate, but the goal remains to engage in activities that result in a healthier brain.

Now add the psychological benefits of exercise, such as stress management and emotional regulation, which both promote healthy coping and overall well-being. Exercise can also benefit your body image and self-confidence, and, if it has a social element, you can build your circle of friends and feel connected to a larger community. So you can live longer, stronger, smarter, healthier, and happier, *and* feel great in your favorite outfit. Are you in yet?

Exercise and Pain

Let's look at what we know about the power of exercise to improve your pain. Here, too, many studies show that exercise helps reduce the severity of pain, improve pain-related functioning, and diminish negative thoughts and emotions that can make pain worse.[44] Exercise training can increase your threshold for pain and can be more effective than other treatments for improving sensitivity to pain, both processes for top-down pain.[45]

It should come as no surprise that exercise represents a first-line therapy for people with chronic pain. The best results require consistency over time, but a meta-analysis found that even a single aerobic or resistance training session could reduce pain sensitivity in healthy individuals.[46] A different meta-analysis considered fifty studies that evaluated more than 3,500 people with chronic pain and found differences in the best type of exercise for top-down pain (fibromyalgia, chronic low back pain) versus bottom-up (rheumatoid arthritis, lupus). The meta-analytic study determined that combining aerobic exercise with strengthening exercise worked better for people with top-down pain than just stretching and flexibility exercises alone.[47]

Yet another recent study of people with chronic pain from osteoar-thritis of the knee found that participating in a regular exercise program improved pain severity and negative thoughts in a way that correlated with changes in activating the prefrontal cortex, the part of the brain responsible for planning and setting goals.[48] This finding indicates that pain improve-ment may be due, at least in part, to exercise-induced changes in the brain. I hope you exercise already. If you don't, I'm trying *very hard* to get you on board. If I'm succeeding, you might be wondering, *OK, what next?*

Find Something That Makes Sense to You

If you're not now or never were an exercise enthusiast, you may dread the thought of going to the gym. That's OK! The good news is that research shows that you have many ways to derive meaningful benefits from exer-cise. Studies reporting benefits for people with pain have tested formal, instructor-led programs that meet a few times a week, walking programs, and even belly dancing. Granted, the belly dancing study was small, but it sounds like fun—and that's the point! Exercise needs to be fun or at least engaging or challenging in a good way to make it feel rewarding. If you're a people person, make it social. If you're a lone wolf, go solo.

Where to Start?

Incorporate a little aerobic exercise, strength training, and flexibility exercise into your long-term Thriving Plan. Aerobic exercise promotes cardiovascular health, immune system functioning, increased energy, healthy sleep, elevated mood, and the list goes on. To reap those benefits while skipping the gym, you can choose from a vast array of *low-impact* classes offered online for all levels and concerns. You also can cycle (a stationary bike counts!), swim, dance, row, and even (or especially) walk briskly. More about walking in a bit. Whatever you choose, you may want to *avoid high-impact aerobic exercise* such as running, jumping, and the rapid lifting and throwing of heavy objects that may take place in a CrossFit class. Low-impact exercise that minimizes stress on your joints is the way to go.

You can do certain yoga classes and circuit training in a way that adequately raises your heart rate. Water-based aerobic exercise reduces impact on joints, increases resistance, and exercising in warm water can feel comforting. Really, the best form of aerobic exercise for you is the one you can do safely, enjoy, and will do regularly.

Exercise to increase strength and flexibility is equally important. Strength training uses resistance (weights, machines, bands) to help build muscle mass. This type of exercise helps reduce bone loss that comes with aging and osteoporosis. In contrast, flexibility exercise increases range of motion, reduces stiffness, and decreases the risk of future injury or re-injury. Flexibility programs typically involve a brief warm-up period to loosen up and then a series of stretches. The movements *should not* cause discomfort. Strength and flexibility programs that use isometric exercises such as yoga, tai chi, and qigong generally help people with chronic pain.

The Benefits of Mind-Body Exercise

Yoga could be the perfect exercise for people with chronic pain but only if led by an expert instructor who can tailor the class to your specific needs. Yoga involves moving your body gently into various positions or poses with the goals of enhancing fitness and flexibility, improving breathing, and relaxing the mind. A meta-analysis by a research team in China showed that yoga for people with chronic low back pain resulted in less pain in the short-term and improved functioning both in the short- and long-term. The study also showed that yoga was as effective as other forms of exercise *and* physical therapy for improving pain, functioning, and quality of life.[49]

Dance Therapy

Dance Therapy, which promotes physical and emotional health, requires a trained therapist to lead the classes. Distinct from dance therapy, aerobic dance classes can include Zumba, Salsa, Jazzercise, and Barre. They haven't undergone extensive study, though, so it's hard to say much about their safety or effectiveness. For some, dance therapy might be fun, social, distracting, and mood-elevating. For others, certain movements may not be appropriate. As with any exercise program, consult your physician before giving them a try.

Walking Works

For people with chronic pain, walking can be just as effective as other forms of exercise. Yes, you read that correctly. If your exercise regimen entails increasing your step count day after day, I'd be happy as a clam for you. Carla Vanti and her colleagues at the University of Bologna conducted a meta-analysis of randomized controlled trials that evaluated the benefits of walking versus other types of exercise for people with chronic low back pain. They found that pain, disability, fear avoidance, and quality of life all similarly improved either with walking or other types of exercise.[50] It's *all* good.

You can incorporate walking into your life in so many fun ways. Walk in different parks around your town. Walk your dog an extra 15 minutes a day than normal. Take a nature hike with a friend. Mall walking is great during bad weather and for making new friends. My own favorite is golf. Nothing feels more glorious to me than walking down scenic fairways, wildflowers in bloom, birds singing, furry critters frolicking along the tree line. Even if you don't know how to golf, you likely know or love people who do. If they are walkers, tag along for a round sometime. I'm sure they'll appreciate your keen observations and clever commentary about their golf swings.

What about Physical Therapy? Yes, Yes, Yes!

Physical therapy (PT) is an excellent place to start if you haven't exercised in a long time, never had an evaluation for the best exercise for you, or have pain from an injury. Numerous studies conducted on people with chronic pain have shown robust benefits for PT, especially increased functioning. PT also tends to be highly personalized, another big positive. A physical therapist evaluates your medical history, abilities, and needs, then develops an exercise program to improve your range of motion, strength, and cardiovascular health. PT treatment can also include massage, ice or heat therapy, electrical stimulation techniques, joint mobilization, and others.

Manual physical therapy uses hands-on techniques instead of devices or machines. A study led by Kylie Isenburg at Harvard Medical School showed that manual therapy reduced pain and resulted in changed brain activity in areas associated with cognitive, emotional, and sensory processing of pain.[51] Whatever approach your physical therapist recommends, a more long-term plan typically will consist of regular exercise to maintain your improvements. Ideally your exercise program will consist of aerobic activity and exercise that improves strength, flexibility, and balance.

Exercise? Hello, I Have Chronic Pain!

OK, let's face the dragon in the room. Some days, you simply won't be able to do the exercise you had planned because of a pain flare. That's understandable. Don't feel guilty. On a bad day, you might be able to walk a little and/or stretch stiff and achy muscles for a few minutes. A slow walk in the sunshine or a gentle stretch could make you feel a little or a lot better.

For now, start by picking *anything* that sounds like fun and give it a try. If you need to adapt your expectations to meet your level of fitness, ability to move, and pain on any given day, that's OK. The goal is to move a little each day, move a bit more the next day, and the day after that. Gauge your progress with a fitness app on your smartphone or a dedicated tracker such as a pedometer or Fitbit. It feels amazingly satisfying to meet and even exceed your daily step goal.

Also set reasonable goals, especially at first. They should be easily reachable. You can increase them incrementally over time. Pair up with a friend or family member as an exercise buddy who will encourage you, hold you accountable, offer social support, and make the time pass more pleasantly.

Good Days and Bad

Most people with chronic pain report having some good days. Your pain feels better and perhaps you have a bit more energy, right? As a result, you attempt every line item on your to-do list. That rarely turns out well, does it? You probably can attest to falling into the trap of overdoing it on a good day only to be wiped out for *days* afterward with a serious pain flare. It feels even more depressing when you figure out that you might have done as much or more over the same number of days if you had taken it easy and not triggered that pesky flare.

The better strategy is to take care of your normal tasks. Relish that you feel OK and maybe do *one* more activity that you enjoy. It's hard to remember not to overdo it on good days. But it's even harder to do anything on the days you feel lousy. On those bad days try to do one small activity that you enjoy in a wise and gentle manner.

Time-Based Activity Pacing

If you've fallen into the trap of doing too much on good days more than a few times, try a strategy like time-based activity pacing. This strategy works better for starting a new exercise program rather than trying to complete a full class or specific number of minutes of activity while pushing through the pain. Time-based pacing alternates periods of activity with periods of rest. You do an activity, say an exercise, for a safe and set amount of time. You predetermine the amount of time that you can do it safely without making your pain worse, then you take a break for a number of minutes that you also predetermine and repeat until you achieve your total goal.

Let's say your exercise program consists of brisk walking in the park, and you know that you can walk briskly for ten minutes without causing a pain flare. Begin your pacing by walking briskly for those ten minutes. Then walk slowly or sit for, say, five minutes, then start the cycle of brisk walking for ten minutes followed by five minutes of rest. Repeat the pattern until you reach your goal for this exercise session. In Part Two of the book, we'll revisit this strategy and apply it to other activities and tasks.

Who Has Time to Exercise?

Yes, people with chronic pain tend to lead hectic lives. If you have zero time for exercise, here's my counteroffer. A strategy called lifestyle activity exercise simply means supercharging your regular daily activities. You probably have heard of this before. Take the stairs instead of the escalator or elevator. Walk or bike to work. Do your standard chores in double time. It might sound a little silly, but it works. Do what you normally do while increasing your activity level or time. Remember, an activity app or monitor will tell you where you stand—or walk!—and you can circle your living room while watching TV to land those final 500 steps you need for the day.

———

Whatever you do, make exercise something you *want* to do, not something you must do. The key to beating procrastination is excitement. We avoid what we don't want to do in favor of what seems easier or more enjoyable. If your exercise routine feels fun and easy, *voilà*, instant success!

IDEAS TO REMEMBER

- Exercise has numerous benefits for chronic pain, including improving pain severity, flexibility, range of motion, balance, strength, physical functioning, cardiovascular health, emotional health, and brain function.
- If your physician says it's OK, find a form of exercise or physical activity that appeals to you and do it. Swimming, cycling, dancing, yoga, and just walking briskly all count!
- Lifestyle activity counts, too. Do what you normally do, but add extra time, steps, stairs, hills, movements, energy, or speed.
- Physical therapy is a great place to learn the best exercises for you and get you moving safely again.
- Use time-based pacing to plan rigorous physical activities such as shoveling snow, raking leaves, or house cleaning in order to avoid triggering pain flares.

Lived Experience: John

In 2008, I was falling apart and found myself in the hospital, being treated by an addiction specialist. It was a stunning development. Things like that didn't happen to me. I'm a reverend, for goodness' sake! I had followed doctor's orders to take opioids for my pain. Between the opioids and my unrelenting pain, my life started to unravel. Fortunately, the addiction specialist understood my predicament, passed no judgment, and slowly weaned me off the opioids. He also started me on a nonaddictive pain medication that I still take.

My journey with chronic pain began in the spring of 1989, when I developed widespread body pain and received a diagnosis of fibromyalgia. Since then, postherpetic nerve pain, a generous helping of osteoarthritis, and plenty of back pain joined the mix, as well as an impressive daily cocktail of meds. I also have bipolar disorder that leans toward depression, with numerous major bouts over the years.

Not until about 2012 did I put together the most important connection regarding my chronic pain. The more depressed I was, the more pain I experienced. The reverse also held true: the more pain I felt, the more depressed I became. My pain and depression somehow work together to form a nasty brew that increases both far beyond what each could do by itself. I brought this idea to the addiction specialist who, years before, had changed my life for the better. He said I was exactly right. Pain and depression work together synergistically but in a bad way, resulting in greater misery. 1 + 1 = 3 (or more!).

What I regret most is that I had the knowledge, but I didn't act on it. Today, as I look back, I can't believe that I just sat on those critical insights for almost two years before I decided to do something. I already took meds for my depression and pain, and they hugely helped, but they weren't enough. I needed to do more. After a fair amount of research, I accepted that exercise had the greatest potential to help with my pain and depression. I had to become more active and, yes, take responsibility for my own healing.

Next came the hard part: getting off my duff and starting to exercise. I'm no gym guy. Lifting weights, going to spin classes, or doing Zumba aren't for me. I do have dogs, though, and they were looking a little round themselves. So the logical step was to start an exercise program for all of us. The first time I walked the dogs, I felt winded easily and gladly came home after just fifteen minutes—and they felt the same. Every day I walked them a little bit further, though, and today we walk between three and five miles at least four times a week.

The best part? It works! My chronic pain is the best it has ever been. So, walk, you can do it, too, but remember to start low, go slow, and smile as you take charge of your own healing.

Reverend John Deuble is a pain warrior.

10

SOCIAL CONNECTEDNESS

Julianne Holt-Lunstad and her colleagues at Brigham Young University conducted a meta-analysis to evaluate factors most likely to ensure survival.[52] They showed that expected factors, such as healthy body weight, exercising regularly, avoiding excessive alcohol consumption, and treating high blood pressure (if you have it) all strongly predict survival. As you might guess, quitting smoking was by far the most important factor. It decreased risk of death by about half. Another health factor was just as powerful as quitting smoking. Any guesses?

Yup, having strong social relationships also decreased risk of death by about 50 percent. What's more, the authors felt that their findings likely underestimated the protective effect. In the studies they considered for their paper that measured social factors using more comprehensive questionnaires, the protective effect looked much stronger, a more than *90 percent increase in the odds of survival.* Wow.

It's late in the day, and there's almost no one on the beach. It's a little chilly, the wind is whipping, and the ocean is angry but magnificent. I'm nine years old, and my dad and I are walking along the shoreline, no further out than knee-deep. The waves start to look more threatening, so we wade back toward the beach.

About twenty feet out, a giant wave hits us from behind, slamming us into the ground. My chin hurts, and all I can see is cloudy water thick with sand, seaweed, and bubbles. I'm weightless, spinning out of control, unsure whether I'm upside down or right side up. A few seconds pass, and a powerful tug pulls me out to sea. It feels as if I've fallen into the rapids of a river—nothing but water and bubbles, no control, no air, and then, terror. Suddenly, pressure around my wrist and I am yanked free from the silty abyss. It's my dad, out of breath, too, barely able to stand. I sputter and choke and finally breathe. We stagger toward the beach. Safe, I look at him, and I always will remember the panic barely concealed in his eyes but also the relief, gratitude, and love.

We all need people in our lives, family and friends who care about us. We flourish when we have a sense of community and belonging. Why? Because it's hard to survive on our own. We're programmed to be tribal, to affiliate with others, and form strong social bonds. Adversity and threats come in many guises. Without adequate personal resources, they can engulf us completely. That's why we sometimes need someone to metaphorically reach down and pluck us out of the roiling sea before we drown.

Social Ties Matter for Everyday Health

People who report having strong social support tend to have less depression and anxiety, better well-being, and a greater sense of self-worth and self-confidence. They're also more likely to have a healthy body mass index, exercise more, sleep better, smoke less, and have a decreased risk for diseases ranging from cancer to dementia.

Bruce McEwen, the influential cell biologist we met when we explored stress and trauma, proposed two critical factors to help you bounce back after stressful events: adequate coping skills and good social support. Our positive friendships not only lift us up when we feel down, but they also make us happier in general and promote a reassuring sense of belonging.

Positive relationships can encourage healthier behavior, such as eating better and exercising more. A caveat applies, however. The benefits related to
social connection largely tie to *healthy* relationships. With sexually, physically, or emotionally abusive relationships, the health effects become negative: more pain, more disease, higher risk of death.[53]

So, your family, friends, and even neighbors affect your health and well-
being. As part of the famous Framingham Heart Study, James Fowler from
the University of California at San Diego and Nicholas Christakis from
Harvard Medical School cataloged the networks of social relationships for
all study participants, including the happiness and unhappiness of participants and their social connections.[54] The investigators observed clusters
of happy and unhappy people within the network. Their remarkable anal-
yses showed that happiness clustering seemed to result from the spread of
happiness from one person to the next rather than from people with similar levels of happiness or unhappiness clustering together. If a friend who
lives within one mile of you becomes happy, the probability that you will be
happy increases by 25 percent. If your neighbor feels happy, your chances of
feeling the same increase by 34 percent! The authors of the study concluded
that happiness, like health, acts as a collective phenomenon. In other words,
we rise and fall together.

Social Connection Affects the Experience of Pain

Many studies look at the harms of social exclusion, rejection, and ostracism.
They broadly show that social exclusion corresponds with the development
of psychiatric disorders, such as depression and anxiety. These same types
of poor social support also strongly influence the experience of pain. For
example, a meta-analysis by Mark Jensen and his team at the University of
Washington in Seattle reported that across twenty-nine studies in people
with physical disabilities including spinal cord injury, muscular sclerosis,
and limb amputation, perceived social support closely associated with pain
and disability across all conditions.[55]

Researchers often study social exclusion with clever experiments. One
of the most common paradigms used to provoke feelings of exclusion and

rejection is a game called Cyberball. The test subject plays a computerized game of catch with two other players supposedly on computers elsewhere in the world. The game begins with all three players amicably tossing the electronic ball to one another. For at least one of three possible tosses, the test subject receives and tosses the ball to one of the other two players. It all feels fair and inclusive. But then the other two players start excluding the test subject, who receives the ball less and less until almost not at all. It might not seem like this simple computer game would spark feelings of exclusion and rejection, but it really does! Test subjects become frustrated, anxious, sad, and even more sensitive to pain.[56] That's right, when feeling socially excluded, test subjects reported higher levels of pain, became more sensitive to a painful stimulus, and had brain activation patterns reflective of experiencing greater pain.[57] Social exclusion also activates the stress-response system. How about that?

Loneliness represents another potent factor for the experience of pain. FIERCE, a community that we built at the Department of Anesthesiology at the University of Michigan, stands for Female Investigators Engaging in Research that will Change Everything, and it supports women in pain research. Victoria Powell, one of my FIERCE mentees, is a palliative medicine physician long interested in the role of loneliness and health. To explore the possibility that loneliness could contribute to the development of chronic pain, a study that she led used data from the University of Michigan's Health and Retirement Study (HRS). It's a longitudinal panel study, meaning that it follows many people over time to observe changes in their health and what factors could relate to the development of new disease. The HRS consists of surveys of nearly 20,000 people in America who represent the larger US population.

For her study, we analyzed the data of almost 6,000 people aged fifty and older who reported their levels of loneliness for at least two time points and later reported their levels of pain, depression, and fatigue.[58] We found that loneliness strongly predicted the development of pain, fatigue, and depression separately, as well as who would develop all three together. Loneliness had this strong effect even when we considered the impact of living alone or with others, demographic variables such as age, sex, education, economic status, and already having some of the symptoms at baseline. This convincing evidence suggests that loneliness plays at least some role in the development of pain and other related symptoms.

It seems strange that just feeling connected to another person or a group can decrease the experience of pain, but that appears to be the case. Studies show that having a large circle of friends has an association with higher pain tolerance.[59] Other studies show that simply having someone close to you in the room while undergoing a painful medical procedure can reduce pain. Human touch appears even more powerful than the presence of a loved one. Studies exploring handholding while experiencing pain show lower ratings for pain severity and less corresponding pain-related brain activity.[60] The pain-reduction effect increases even more when the person holding the hand is a romantic partner rather than a stranger. Proximity and supportive touch seem to decrease the perceived threat that the pain could pose, and this buffering process reduces the experience of pain *in the brain*.

We All Need a Tribe

According to community psychologist David McMillan, four criteria define a community. First is membership: you feel a sense of belonging to the group or larger community. Second is influence, meaning that you have a sense that you make a difference to the group and the group has some sway over you. The third criterion is integration and a fulfilment of needs, which refers to feeling that other group members will meet your needs. Lastly is a sense of shared emotional connection; in other words, you feel that you share time, space, and similar experiences with one another. We all need community, and ideally you belong to several communities where you feel a strong sense of connection as neighbors, colleagues, spiritual or religious companions, sports fans, hobby buddies, school friends, and even online followers. The possibilities are infinite. If you don't have a strong sense of community, you need to build one, but doing so when you have chronic pain comes with some inherent challenges.

Pain Affects Social Connections

Pain can lead to withdrawal from people and activities that you used to love and enjoy, a very real loss. You may grieve the people you no longer see or the activities you no longer do because your pain gets in the way of social activities. You also may experience excessive social sensitivity that can make your fear of rejection so powerful that you simply don't feel comfortable reaching out. Jennifer Pierce, a social psychologist and another FIERCE mentee, studies the role of social relationships in people with chronic pain. Her work explores the possibility that, at least in part, social processes may drive some chronic pain. Her research considers social sensitivity, a heightened sensitivity to negative social experiences, as another form of general sensory sensitivity. This social sensitivity might be more pronounced in people with pain who have a history of trauma because they already have increased general sensitivity.[61] Traumatic experiences can alter how people view social interactions. They can result in paying too much attention to negative social cues and having more negative evaluations of the intent of others. The brain might detect a threat or bad intentions even when none exists.

Parts of the brain process both social pain, such as distress from social rejection, and physical pain, especially the unpleasantness of pain. This overlap implies that they might share similar threat-detecting alarm systems in the brain, too. Addressing social pain could improve the experience of physical pain and, perhaps, vice versa.

Nathan Dewall and his colleagues at the University of Kentucky had participants take acetaminophen (Tylenol) or a placebo daily for three weeks. In diaries, study participants also logged their impressions of social rejection every day. Dewall and his team found that the people taking acetaminophen reported experiencing less daily social rejection compared to people taking the placebo.[62] The researchers also used neuroimaging to evaluate the brain activity of study participants and found that acetaminophen reduced brain responses to social rejection in regions associated with social distress and the emotional aspects of physical pain. An over-the-counter pain reliever improved the effects of painful social rejection. Whoa!

What Does That Mean for People with Chronic Pain?

For the people with chronic pain at our outpatient clinic, we found that only about half report having strong social support. Many still need to build the powerful sense of community that they deserve. Did you notice how I put the impetus for building these relationships on the person with pain? Strong relationships and a sense of community don't just happen. Relationships need attention, patience, and perseverance. They're hard work but worth it. Several activities in Part Two will target repairing damaged relationships, building stronger relationships, and finding new communities to support your health and happiness.

Do Pets Count?

Yes, to some degree. Studies show that pet ownership corresponds with greater happiness and better health. Of course, the benefits depend largely on the quality of the relationship with your pet. If your pet keeps you awake at night, behaves destructively, or isn't loving, it could cause more harm than benefits. If you already have fur babies—and those of you who do know exactly what I mean—then the benefits are more obvious. Pets can help us feel less lonely, more needed, and provide a safe outlet for emotional expression. The love between you and your critter is real, and it flows two ways.

When dog owners interact with their pups in a caring manner, such as cuddling or sharing loving glances, oxytocin, the bonding hormone, is released. Even more remarkable, dogs release oxytocin in these loving moments with their owners, too. The love flows both ways and, because oxytocin is analgesic, can decrease the experience of pain. In a recent study led by Ben Carey at the University of Saskatchewan in Canada, investigators had emergency room patients interact with a therapy dog or wait as normal for ER care.[63] Patients who spent as little as ten minutes with the therapy dog rated much lower pain severity than the people who just waited.

Pet ownership also has a doubling effect. Not only does having pets offer direct benefits for health and happiness, but studies also show that dog ownership in particular has the added benefits of getting us off the couch and outside for regular walks, providing more opportunities to interact with other people and build more supportive communities. Casual conversations with strangers who ask about our dogs and the comradery of owners mingling at the dog park come to mind. Cats, birds, reptiles, and other pets also can engage other humans in conversation and prompt shared-interest friendships.

Final Thoughts about Social Connections

At the start of this chapter, I shared a story about my dad and me on a stormy beach many years ago. We both were in peril, but he didn't just save himself, which he could have done. Instead, he put himself in further jeopardy to save me. That act goes against a personal survival instinct and good sense. We humans are programmed to care for one another for the good of the tribe, to ensure our survival, to ensure that we thrive as a species. Make building and tending to your circle of friends and family a priority.

In the end, your fondest memories won't be about the work project that caused you to skip a family vacation or the groceries you bought instead of taking a call from a friend whose life was unraveling. You will value most the time you spent with loved ones; the new places you visited and the people you met; the meals you shared; the momentous experiences of births, graduations, and weddings; and the shared moments, both glad and sad, that give our lives meaning. That's what truly matters most.

IDEAS TO REMEMBER

- Humans are social animals. Our need to affiliate helps ensure survival. Strong social relationships predict better mental and physical health, including a reduced risk for most diseases and a decreased risk for death.
- Social support is a key factor for living with pain and disability, yet only about half of people with chronic pain report having strong social support.
- Quality of relationships counts. Good relationships are protective, while toxic relationships increase the risk for poor health.
- It's up to you to build your tribe. You can't always pick your family members, neighbors, or boss, but you can control how you respond to them and with whom you spend your spare time. Build new friendships and strengthen those you value most.

Lived Experience: Shanna

I was twelve years old when I got my first migraine, thirteen when I started to feel intense knee pain, sixteen when I had my first knee surgery, twenty-two when fatigue hit, and twenty-six when my stomach issues began. New diagnoses kept rolling in: chronic migraine, osteoarthritis, fibromyalgia, hip impingements, mast cell activation syndrome, Celiac disease, postural orthostatic tachycardia syndrome, pelvic joint disarrangement. Sometimes chronic illness can feel like playing Pokémon—gotta catch 'em all!

Yet, I'm so lucky to exist as a disabled and chronically ill person in the time that I do. I, like many others in this community, have experienced excessive discrimination due to my disability, isolation, and struggles navigating the US healthcare system; but, I also have found a brilliant community to uplift and care for me. We are stronger together, even when many of us connect from our beds or couches.

About ten years ago, I came across the idea of "spoons" in terms of invisible or nonapparent disabilities. Others who don't know you quickly look you over and "see" that you aren't disabled or chronically ill, which really complicates life at times. Sometimes people yell at me for parking in an accessible space, despite my disability permit. Other times, they glare at me for where I sit on public transportation. People who haven't lived this experience don't understand what it's like to navigate our able-bodied-centered world when you don't look how they expect disabled people to look (using a wheelchair, assistive devices, or a service animal).

The spoons concept comes from Christine Miserandino of ButYou DontLookSick.com, a woman living with lupus. At a diner, a friend asked her to explain the impact of lupus on her life. She picked up a pile of spoons, noting that she started each day with a finite number of them. As she goes through her day, she pulls spoons from the pile based on the amount of energy and capacity a given activity takes. For example, a quick rinse might cost one spoon, while a full shower, plus washing and styling hair, might take three. By the end of the day, she often has only one spoon left and has to decide what to do with it.

Spoon Theory caught on in the disability and chronic illness community. What a phenomenal way to explain our capacity (or lack thereof) in any given moment, to ourselves and our partners, friends, and colleagues. Being able to say, "I'd love to go, but I'm all out of spoons" can land differently than just "I can't go." Sometimes my friends respond in kind, offering to come over to watch movies, which is less demanding than going to a movie theater.

Many of us call ourselves Spoonies, and we connect in many ways. During my time in Colorado, I started a virtual Spoonies group there and have started one here in Michigan. We share resources, such as knowledgeable healthcare providers or suggestions for pain management, and we have a collective space to kvetch about our low-spoon, high-pain days. When we "catch" a new diagnosis to add to our Pokédex, we have space to share, to process, to feel supported by our community. The kindness of and fellowship with these people has made all the difference.

———

Shanna Katz Kattari is associate professor of social work at the University of Michigan, a disability activist, and founder of Michigan Spoonies and Colorado Spoonies.

11

MUST DO VERSUS LOVE TO DO

No matter our health, we all have limited physical and mental resources to do everything we'd like to do in a day. This reality holds particularly true for people with chronic pain, who have just a few precious spoons per day. It can feel so frustrating to run out of gas or experience so much pain that you can't give loved ones the attention and care they need. You might not even have enough energy to take off your shoes before falling into bed, much less drawing that warm bubble bath you envisioned all day. Foregoing what matters most and the critical elements of self-care becomes an all-too-common problem for people with chronic illnesses.

Compound that with trying to do too much on the days that you do feel good. Remember that glorious morning when you woke with more energy and less pain. You instantly thought about making up for lost time, trying to run *all* your errands, getting a little exercise, and catching up on socializing *all in the same day*. You know how that works out in the end. Studies that track the relationship between daily activity and chronic pain symptoms have shown that an overly taxing day can result in a pain flare that lasts for several days afterward. The surge of activity to catch up sets you back further because you must spend more time recovering, doing literally nothing.

This exhausting cycle of too much activity on good days and no activity on bad days isn't the answer.

Instead, try to find a balance between doing what you must and doing what you enjoy. Also try to engage in a consistent level of activity every day. This means that you'll have slight upticks and slight downticks in your activity levels, based on how you feel, but aim for minimal variability from day to day. Picture a scale of one to ten, with one representing no activity and ten the maximum. You want to avoid swinging from an eight to a two. The better strategy is to plan your activity levels to range from four to six each day, good or bad. On bad days, maintain some activity, even if you need to adapt tasks to make them more manageable. Similarly, on good days, don't overdo it; perhaps do only a wee bit more than you normally would.

Valued Activities Make Life More Rewarding

The concept of valued life activities (VLAs) in people with chronic pain comes from the pioneering work of Lois Verbrugge.[64] With conditions as disabling as rheumatoid arthritis was before the creation of new classes of drugs, clinicians and researchers mostly evaluated "instrumental" activities, such as bathing, dressing, and preparing meals, and "committed" activities, including going to work, running errands, and doing chores around the house. But with better medications came a focus on "discretionary" activities, enjoyable leisure pursuits, which can be even more important for the general health and well-being of people with chronic illness.

The importance of discretionary activities inspired Patricia Katz and Ed Yellen to explore the impact of chronic illness and pain on VLAs. VLAs give life joy and meaning and can include just about anything: participating in sports, such as tennis, golf, or swimming; playing a musical instrument, singing in a choir, or dancing; engaging in hobbies; traveling; or socializing with friends and family. Research conducted by Katz and Yellen followed people with rheumatoid arthritis over time and found that the illness-related loss of VLAs reliably predicted the onset of depression. They found that not being able to do VLAs resulted in having almost six times the odds of developing depression![65] A very large body of research shows that the more depressed someone feels, the worse almost every chronic illness becomes, and quality of life plummets.

What does that mean for you? A crucial element of your chronic pain reset and Thriving Plan is to do at least one personally meaningful activity—or one that simply makes you happy—every day. No matter how lousy you feel, commit to one positive action. It could be anything as long as it makes you smile, feels rewarding, or functions as a building block for a better future. On good days, you likely will engage in the activity more fully, making it feel even more gratifying. Then, on bad days, you can recall that good action and reflect that the day wasn't a total loss. I hope you will commit to adding more VLAs to all your days, good and bad. Let's look at some strategies for how to do so more successfully.

Scheduling Pleasant Activities Makes Happiness a Priority

If, during your next healthcare visit, your provider said: "I'm prescribing that you take time to have some fun." You probably would think they're joking or in serious need of a vacation, but you'd be wrong. Many studies show that when people feel happier, they live longer lives, engage in more health-promoting behaviors, and generally have better disease outcomes, meaning less disability, less severe symptoms, less time recovering from illness, and so on. Those findings hold especially true for people with chronic pain.

The strategy of scheduling pleasant activities initially was used to help people with depression, but it's also a potent technique for people with chronic pain. Both depression and living with chronic pain can lead to withdrawal and inactivity. When we withdraw, we alienate the social support we need most when we feel down. Inactivity typically results in muscle deconditioning—and weak muscles tend to ache more!—along with the absence of the mood-boosting benefits of exercise and activity. Over time, a downward spiral of withdrawal and inactivity leads to increasing misery. That's not good for anyone.

While scheduling pleasant activities has not been as well studied in chronic pain, a meta-analysis that considered sixteen studies examining the effectiveness of this intervention in people with depression found strikingly robust benefits.[66] Other meta-analyses assessing the effectiveness of antidepressant medication found an effect size of 0.30 (small benefits).[67] The effect size for scheduling positive activities was 0.87—very large (big benefits)! Antidepressants certainly can help but scheduling pleasant activities, when added to your existing care, might be able to help even more.

By scheduling pleasant activities, you create a social contract with yourself to do something you love, at an appointed time, without excuses for why the action should wait or yield to an obligatory activity (chores, errands). I'm excited for you to give this a try in the second part of this book!

Doing What You Love Creates Positive Emotions

Willingness to expend precious energy on VLAs by making time for them during your daily routine is step one. Engaging in absorbing activities that you love improves the number, type, and intensity of positive emotions, which in turn help buffer the harmful effects of stress and negative emotions. When you do what you love, you tend to feel more hopeful, connected, happy, calm, competent, and all sorts of other good stuff. As Barbara Fredrickson from the University of North Carolina has shown in her groundbreaking research, positive emotions can create an *upward* spiral, meaning that the better you feel, the more you do, and better things seem to come your way.[68] Happy, engaged people draw others to them like bees to a flower. The more you build your social circle, the more connected you feel, and better health and happiness will follow. Amazing!

Doing What You Love Creates More Flow

If you have heard about Mihaly Csikszentmihalyi, you probably know about the notion of *flow*. (Yeah, I can't pronounce his name either.)[69] In his book *Flow: The Psychology of Optimal Experience*, Csikszentmihalyi proposed that, for athletes, musicians, and gamers, flow is known as being "in the zone." It involves deep focus and energy, and time seems not to exist. You feel mindful, present, and tuned into the activity, experiencing a sense of challenge, perhaps on the cusp of impending success. This state feels like nothing else, when time and place melt away, and only what you're doing exists.

Being in a state of flow has numerous benefits. In a decade-long longitudinal study, Susie Cranston and Scott Keller found that, when people were performing in flow states, they were 500 percent more productive.[70] Wow, think what you could accomplish in just a small amount of time when in a state of flow! When experiencing flow, pain often feels miles away. Flow represents the ultimate distraction, thus buffering the experience of pain, likely by affecting brain function. It's a lot like being in a meditative state, and we already noted the health benefits of meditation: improved mood and less stress, inflammation, and muscle tension.

Doing What You Love Can Be Hard or Impossible with Chronic Pain

For many with chronic pain, certain activities are just too demanding, especially with some sports. Yet a study that considered the results from more than 120 studies of exercise with chronic low back pain, researchers concluded that swimming, walking, and cycling—when practiced at moderate intensity—helped maintain fitness and improved pain. Other sports, such as tennis, golf, and martial arts, performed at a lower intensity, also helped. Investigators did caution against ball sports, including football, basketball, and soccer, for obvious reasons.[71] If your physician says a particular sport or other activity is OK for you, schedule it, adapt it, and pace it accordingly.

Adapting an activity just means changing how you do it so you *can* do it. You might do it more slowly; with different equipment, tools, or assistive devices; or in a less competitive setting. You might have to omit parts of it or change them dramatically. Look at the activity with a critical eye, go easy on yourself, and decide what's reasonable. Let's say you love golf, but your clubs are gathering dust. A first step could be grabbing your wedge and a putter and practicing your short game just once a week at first. Next, you might try some half swings with a nine iron at the driving range. It feels good to see the ball fly a bit, right? Maybe join friends on a nine-hole outing, use a cart, and just play the short game. Walk when you can and pitch in from fewer than fifty yards. Even if you've never touched a golf club, you get the point: *start low* (doing the minimum by adapting the activity) and *go slow* (slowly increasing your activity level over time).

Pacing an activity just means not overdoing it. As you begin a new activity, it's better to do a little less than a little more. Never let pain be your guide. In other words, stop doing what you're doing *before* it hurts too much. Instead, do the activity for a safe amount of time, then rest for a bit. After resting, you might feel like you can do the activity again for the same amount of time, then rest once again. Never push yourself to finish something only for the sake of finishing it. We'll try activity pacing based on time in Part Two of the book.

I Don't Have Time!

Well, maybe you do. Our electronic devices, like black holes, suck up our precious free moments. The average adult in America spends about 195 hours a year on social media. Facebook users spend even more time: 297 hours a year![72] Then consider total screen time across all your devices and related activities (work, TV, gaming, texting, email). Some estimates place total daily screen time as high as seventeen hours per day![73]

How time-consuming is your device use? Check your usage stats on the device, if available, or try keeping a device diary for three days. Log how much time you spend in front of a screen, any screen, working, watching TV, on social media, texting, shopping, gaming, etc., then add it all up. If, after your three-day experiment, you don't like the number of screen hours that you logged, consider a one-day device holiday. At the end of an e-free day, note how you feel. Did you feel like you had more time? I bet you did! How was your mood? Hopefully it's great because, instead of staring at a screen, you went for a pleasant walk or connected with a good friend in person.

Yes, I hear you. On bad days, our devices keep us connected and entertained. But really, how do you feel after a couple of hours doom scrolling on social media? Is your pain ever better afterward? Also, ask yourself what else would feel more rewarding, help you build your future, or improve how you feel right now. Do that VLA instead, modified to accommodate how you feel that day. There's no time better to do what you love than right now. Seriously, put down this book and go have some fun, but please come back tomorrow!

IDEAS TO REMEMBER

- Develop a balance between necessary tasks (work, errands, chores) and enjoyable activities (the stuff that's pleasant and gives your life meaning).
- Aim to engage in a consistent level of activity every day, even when you feel terrible *or* surprisingly good.
- Withdrawal and inactivity lead to misery. The worse you feel, the more you tend to withdraw and become inactive, resulting in a downward spiral.
- A state of flow, when we do what we love and feel deeply immersed in that activity, it's good for brain and body, a bit like meditation.
- When you undertake any activity or exercise, *start low* and *go slow.*

Lived Experience: Cynthia

When I was eight and Daddy jumped off a bridge, I lost him forever and didn't know if I'd ever feel safe again. Shortly after, I made a promise to him: I would earn my college degree, because we often talked about those special years to come. Through that promise, I stayed connected to the man I loved most.

I adored my daddy, who in some ways was just a big kid. He used to take me to Fairyland, where we ate pink popcorn and giggled together riding The Fireball. To this day, I've never seen anyone get as excited about spotting a bear as he did in Yosemite. I loved to hear him bellow when he squeezed my snot-nosed doll's tummy, sending a yellow balloon out her nostril. All this from a man who earned his PhD from MIT.

But there was the other daddy, preoccupied and glassy-eyed. I once brought him an egg my duck laid, thinking he'd be excited to fry it. Instead, he put it in the refrigerator and, without a glance in my direction, went back to making breakfast. I feared I was losing him. Years after his suicide, I learned that he suffered from paranoid schizophrenia.

When my college years came, only my promise mattered. As a singer, dancer, and actor who lived to perform, I didn't need a degree. Still, I attended the University of California at Irvine as a dance major to stay connected to, indeed, stay safe with Dad's memory. In ballet class, I sustained the injury that triggered my complex regional pain syndrome (CRPS), a disease that forced me to leave school just before graduation. It soon progressed to the point that I was bedridden for a decade and unable to speak for five of those years.

The devastation of CRPS took everything I held dear: my career, my independence, my ability to get married and have a child. Through the never-ending pain that made me feel like I'd been doused with gasoline and lit on fire, I never questioned that I would go back and finish my degree. Once I was well enough to use a wheelchair and run a nonprofit to help other women in pain, I regularly reached out to Irvine administrators, requesting to return. Despite a series of negative replies pouring in, a state senator and I appealed to the school's chancellor. He responded: "Cynthia will never be allowed to earn her degree from UC Irvine," adding that "the dance faculty voted against her chance to return."

That deeply angered me. I refuse to be a victim, and I see every "no" as a future "yes." I reached out to a trusted colleague, a major fundraiser for UC Santa Barbara, and he shared my plight with a UC regent and former ambassador to Yemen. This angel of a woman knew exactly which button to push. I quickly heard from the dean of UC Irvine's dance department, detailing the steps to my diploma.

This prompted an invitation to speak to UC Irvine's injury prevention class. Surrounded by a bevy of dewy-eyed ballerinas, I shared my cautionary tale, adding that I'd be receiving my dance degree from my wheelchair, right alongside them, twenty-three years late. They clapped, screamed, and thumped their toe shoes on the floor. This was in the same studio where I'd suffered the injury.

Earning my dance degree was the proudest moment of my life. As I rolled into that hall, I was radiant knowing that I had kept my promise, certain that Daddy was looking down on me, happy and proud. I was saved.

————

Cynthia Toussaint is an author and founder of For Grace, a not-for-profit organization devoted to promoting better care and wellness for women in pain. Learn more at ForGrace.org.

12

VALUES, VIRTUES, AND STRENGTHS

Cynthia Toussaint's tremendous strength and resiliency helped her succeed in life despite childhood trauma and seemingly overwhelming obstacles. What helped her do that? Think about it. What comes to mind? Courage, hope, perseverance, even zest. A woman of high character, she lives life according to her values. Tapping into your own unique mix of character strengths will make you better able to put your values into action and lead a life that feels more meaningful and rewarding.

Character matters. We all hope to work for fair employers who demonstrate good leadership. For those of us who have them, we strive to raise children who grow up to be honest, kind adults who find loyal and loving partners. We feel the most comfortable and happy when we behave in ways that reflect our values and best character. Our deepest values inform our judgments about our character and the character of others. Succinctly put, your character strengths help make you your best you. Knowing those strengths, putting them to work daily, and discovering new ways to capitalize on them greatly increases your odds of feeling successful in life. Living in accordance with your values makes life feel more purposeful and coherent, key markers for happiness. Contemporary science finally is catching up to Heraclitus, the ancient Greek philosopher who reportedly said: "Character is destiny."

On the other side of the coin, psychology and psychiatry traditionally have focused on diagnosing and treating what goes wrong with the human psyche and human behavior. We're a fallible lot, that's for sure! Nonetheless, we're more than our faults and foibles. We also have the capacity for great good. The field of positive psychology acknowledges our complexities and proposes that studying human strengths, happiness, and leading a good life is just as important as studying what can go wrong.

The founders of positive psychology—including Martin Seligman, Chris Peterson, Nansook Park, and Mike Csikszentmihalyi, among many others—explored the human desire to develop and promote good character. In a years long pursuit of this question, they discovered a universal agreement across philosophical and religious traditions, including Christianity, Hinduism, Buddhism, Confucianism, Taoism, Judaism, and Islam, regarding what constitutes moral behavior and a good life. They identified six core virtues: wisdom, humanity, courage, justice, temperance, and transcendence.[74]

Within that framework, they created a classification system not unlike the one used traditionally to categorize psychiatric disorders. Under the six virtues, they pinpointed twenty-four character strengths. *Character Strengths and Virtues: A Handbook and Classification* serves as the manual of good mental health and human resilience.[75] It carefully describes the process of arriving at these specific strengths, providing a blueprint for understanding each as well as how to nurture these strengths in ways to improve our lives.

The descriptions that follow pull from that handbook and the VIA (Values in Action) Institute on Character, a not-for-profit organization dedicated to the assessment and study of character. As you read through the descriptions, take mental notes of the virtues that you value most and the character strengths you already possess. We all have at least a little of all the strengths, but look for the five or so strengths that resonate most with you. Circle or color in the stars denoting those strengths. I've also included ideas about new ways you can use your specific character strengths (and others) that could help you lead a more rewarding life despite the pain. Remember, we all have a unique combination of strengths; don't be shy, own your strengths. Your unique combination of strengths should be identified and nurtured to help you put your values into action and be your true best self.

Wisdom

This virtue focuses on cognitive strengths that relate to your interest in and tendency toward building knowledge.

☆ CREATIVITY   This strength refers to using new ways to think about or do something that makes a positive contribution. It can include artistic pursuits but isn't limited to them. If you continually look for ways to beautify your home, garden, or yard, use that same creativity to brainstorm hacks for making what you love to do doable again.

☆ CURIOSITY   Having an innate fascination about new ideas, people, places, or experiences and a strong desire to learn more about them characterizes this strength. If you often find yourself falling down Wiki-holes, use that natural curiosity about how the world works to understand how the brain processes pain and ways to help reset it.

☆ OPEN-MINDEDNESS   This strength means using critical thinking, good judgment, and psychological flexibility when drawing conclusions. When presented with new information, you absorb it and update your thinking. If you use this strength to get along with family members, turn it inward to deflect self-criticism and to change how you think about your pain.

☆ LOVE OF LEARNING   Like curiosity, love of learning focuses on systematically adding to what you know already. If you used this strength to master a second language or to read the complete works of a favorite author, use it to dig deeper into developing new skills to manage your pain better.

☆ PERSPECTIVE   Having perspective means you can see the big picture. You learn from mistakes and give great advice. If you often help friends and loved ones make better decisions, think about the next phase of your life in the same way: filled with great possibilities.

Humanity

This virtue relates to enhancing your relationships with others.

☆ KINDNESS   Research shows that kindness, or the tendency to behave considerately of others, correlates with healthy relationships and greater happiness. If you typically take care of everyone else around you, focus on being kind to yourself, for example: forgiving yourself for something that makes you feel bad or engaging in self-care.

☆ LOVE   This strength refers less to the emotion and more to the act of valuing close relationships and genuinely expressing a corresponding sense of connection. If you show your love by supporting a significant other or child who feels sick, lonely, or down, turn those acts of compassion inward to support yourself in similar ways.

☆ SOCIAL INTELLIGENCE   Also known as emotional intelligence, this strength means having an awareness of others' motives and feelings. If you easily lead a team of diverse people with differing agendas, use this strength to help others understand your limitations—and strengths!

Courage

This category helps you face adversity and bounce back, a particularly important virtue for resiliency.

☆ BRAVERY   This strength doesn't imply the absence of fear but denotes not shrinking from a threat, challenge, or pain, *despite* fear. If you use bravery to try physical activities that might prove to be painful, channel that bravery to make a few new friends.

☆ HONESTY OR INTEGRITY　Speaking the truth, acting with honor, and taking responsibility for actions and emotions characterize this strength. If you typically use your integrity in the workplace, honestly explore emotions that you tend to avoid and thoughts that make you uncomfortable. Remember, they're only thoughts and feelings, and you never have to act on them.

☆ PERSEVERANCE　This strength encompasses the persistence to finish what you started, despite obstacles that include time. It can be helpful for learning new skills, enhancing abilities, and improving other strengths. If you persevere at household chores or work duties, apply your perseverance to pursuing activities that bring you joy.

☆ ZEST　Woohoo! Zest is all about living life wholeheartedly, with great enthusiasm and a sense of adventure. Strongly related to emotional and physical health, zest represents one of the most important strengths to build to make your life more active and rewarding. If you engage in your favorite hobby with zest, direct that zeal to more mundane tasks in ways that make each day count.

Justice

This virtue promotes successful interactions with others in groups, for example, at work, in your neighborhood, or the broader community.

☆ FAIRNESS　This strength describes the tendency to treat all people equitably without letting personal feelings bias how you act. Everyone gets a fair chance. If you pride yourself on treating others fairly, turn that strength inward and treat yourself with greater fairness and less harsh judgment.

☆ LEADERSHIP　Successfully encouraging a group to reach its goals while supporting good relations among its members constitutes good leadership. If you display strong leadership in the workplace, apply those same skills at home. Approaching loved ones with more tact, support, and patience will help them and perhaps inspire them to do the same with you.

☆ TEAMWORK OR CITIZENSHIP   This strength refers to working well as a member of a group, small or large. It requires loyalty and a willingness to contribute to the greater good. If you use this strength to complete tasks at home with family members, try your hand at volunteering, for example to restore a public park or establish a community garden.

Temperance

This virtue helps you manage your impulses and keeps you grounded.

☆ FORGIVENESS   This strength refers to being accepting of the shortcomings of others in a merciful way. It doesn't mean condoning or encouraging bad behavior in others, but it does free you from the destructive forces of resentment and hate. If you use forgiveness to smooth family relationships, try forgiving yourself instead of holding yourself to impossibly high standards.

☆ HUMILITY   Humble people don't see themselves as more special than others, but they also aren't self-critical. Let accomplishments speak for themselves. If you use this strength to model good behavior for children, try using it to seek feedback at work or from your closest friends.

☆ PRUDENCE   This strength denotes exerting due care when making decisions or generally showing restraint. Prudent people don't take unwarranted risks or engage in hasty actions that might lead to regret. If you exhibit prudence when making big decisions, such as changing jobs or buying a home, use prudence to not overdo it on a good day.

☆ SELF-REGULATION   Regulating yourself means controlling how you act and feel, using self-discipline to control urges, emotions, and appetites. If you self-regulate to watch what you eat, channel that power the next time you feel upset to quell your emotions by taking three deep breaths.

Transcendence

This virtue touches on your spiritual self and helps create meaning in life.

☆ APPRECIATION OF BEAUTY AND EXCELLENCE   Beauty presents in many forms: art, dance, literature, music, and nature, to name just a few. If you employ this strength to enjoy a whirl around the museum, open yourself to the beauty of a walk in your local park. Seek beauty in the ordinary, and it will become *extraordinary.*

☆ GRATITUDE   This strength is one of the most important for physical and emotional health. It refers to an awareness of and thankfulness for all the good in your life. If you often express gratitude in the context of a spiritual practice, articulate it to people who could benefit from hearing your appreciation.

☆ HOPE   More than just wanting the best to happen, hope entails doing the work to help make it happen. The process includes positive expectations, optimistic thinking, *and* purposeful planning. This strength isn't passive; it involves *action.* If you use hope to dream of a pain-free future, channel it into one small action, each day, to get you there.

☆ HUMOR   Laughter with others promotes bonding and can help ease emotional and physical pain. This strength also includes playfulness and the willingness to appreciate the unexpected in light of difficult circumstances. If you like to crack wise to break the ice in tense situations, try using humor to distract yourself strategically on days when your pain feels worse.

☆ SPIRITUALITY   This strength includes a sense of faith, purpose, or connectedness. Having anchoring beliefs about life and your role in it can guide your behavior and bring you comfort. If you rely on your spirituality to help you weather adversity, tap into your spirituality when feeling happy and embrace gratitude and awe.

Character Strengths in People with Chronic Pain

What strengths sounded like you? Go back, look at the headers again. Did you star a few of them? If not, please do so now.

You might wonder how those strengths matter to people with chronic pain and whether certain strengths can help more than others. In a series of studies in people with chronic pain led by Marianna Graziosi and her team at the University of Pennsylvania and Ryan Niemiec from the VIA Institute on Character, they evaluated strengths with the goal of improving pain self-efficacy—meaning the belief that you can function well, despite your pain.[76] People with high levels of pain self-efficacy tend to have better health-related quality of life, including good sleep and functioning. For the first study, which surveyed 491 people with chronic pain, questionnaires assessed the character strengths most associated with good pain self-efficacy. They found that zest and perseverance were associated with the highest levels of pain self-efficacy.

In another study, they randomly assigned 122 people with chronic pain to one of four groups tasked with writing activities intended to build a particular strength: group one for improving zest, group two for improving leadership, group three for improving spirituality, and a control group to write about the participants' personality. Results again pointed to zest as the most promising strength to boost pain self-efficacy.

In a third study, eighty-one people with chronic pain either wrote about what they did during the day (the control group) or wrote about how they used zest each day. You guessed it. This third study replicated the key findings from the second study, showing that improving zest significantly improved pain self-efficacy. Keep reading for a version of that activity that you can try yourself.

In a recent clinical trial conducted at the CPFRC, we used the Brief Strengths Test to evaluate 100 people with chronic pain. We found that the most common strengths in people with chronic pain included: honesty, kindness, creativity, humor, and love of learning. Like most studies looking at varied populations, prudence and self-regulation ranked low. But unique to chronic pain, the least common strength was (*drum roll, please*) . . . zest. Those 100 people, who each endorsed seven or eight strengths, selected zest only seven times. Now, just because a strength falls low on the list, that doesn't mean it's a weakness. Think of it as a growth area.

Signature Strengths Endorsed

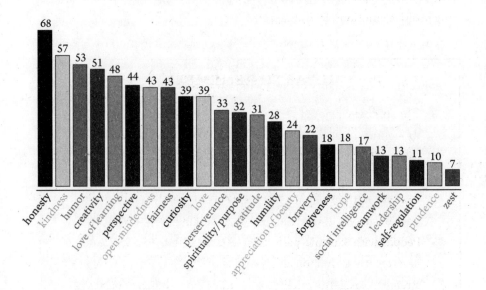

Try This Zest Test

Let's define zest this way. You have enthusiasm for life. You feel highly energetic and activated. You use your energy to the fullest degree.

Here is your assignment: For the next two weeks, try to add a little zest into at least one activity each day. At the end of the day, write a sentence or two about how you used zest that day. That's it!

What Are Your Character Strengths?

Selecting the strengths that you think you possess turns out to be pretty accurate when compared to formal, validated questionnaires, but also consider taking the free survey available on the website for the VIA Institute on Character (VIACharacter.org). More than 20 million people have taken the survey, which offers a free, downloadable PDF of your results. As you try the activities in the second part of the book, think about flexing your top strengths and building those that are important to you but appear lower on the list. You'll find that many of the activities in Part Two focus on improving positive emotions, including zest.

IDEAS TO REMEMBER

- The six core virtues of positive psychology are wisdom, humanity, courage, justice, temperance, and transcendence, and those categories consist of twenty-four character strengths.
- Your strengths can make you the best possible you. Knowing your strengths and putting them to work greatly increases the odds of success at whatever you do, including decreasing pain.
- People with chronic pain most often exhibit honesty, kindness, creativity, humor, and love of learning. The least common strength was zest, which other studies have shown is particularly important for people with pain.
- As part of your Thriving Plan, consider defining your values, embracing your strengths, and enhancing zest to help you lead a better life.

13

GRIT, GRATITUDE, AND GRACE

As tracer rounds whizzed over their heads and ordinance exploded close enough to shake the ground, Liam wondered for the 500th time, *What the hell am I doing here?* He was what you might call a nontraditional basic training soldier. At age thirty-three, with creaky knees and a degree in forestry from the University of Montana, he no longer could resist the voice beckoning him to military service since he was a kid. Now, sitting in a deep trench in the dark with men and women almost half his age and surveying a controlled but still dangerous combat-simulation exercise, he turned to his battle buddies.

"Let's do this," he said with more conviction than he felt, before they launched into the smoky fray. Crawling on their bellies with their faces in the sand, they crossed the wet open field. Along the way, they negotiated barbed wire, logs, and other obstacles as explosions thundered and phosphorus flares lit the night sky. At the end of their journey, a tap on the helmet from above and a hand offered to pull him out of the muck signaled that he completed the last task of training. All current members of Delta Company now qualified for graduation. As always, some who started with the company couldn't withstand the physical, emotional, social, and mental challenges of basic training that test, bend, and build the remarkable young men and women who volunteer to protect our country. *Hooah!* Liam is my son.

Identifying the factors that lead people to drop out or wash out from basic training remains a critical question for the US military. It costs a lot to train new recruits, especially at the highest levels, such as soldiers accepted to the Military Academy at West Point. Despite rigorous application requirements—including a recommendation from a member of Congress—close to one in twenty cadets, when subjected to the early training period called Beast Barracks, drop out in the first summer.

True Grit

Two studies by Angela Duckworth at the University of Pennsylvania explored personality factors that might predict completion of training at West Point.[77] She and her colleagues evaluated nearly 2,500 cadets by means of questionnaires administered soon after arriving at the academy, along with their military records. The researchers found that one psychological factor best predicted who would withstand that first difficult summer: grit, defined as the passion for and healthy perseverence toward long-term achievement with little concern for recognition along the way. The investigators concluded that achieving difficult goals requires more than just talent; it also requires sustained, focused application of effort over time. Passion—caring deeply about or valuing something enough to withstand doubt, fear, setbacks, pain, and exhaustion—often drives this sustained effort.

It seems logical that grit could help people live more successfully with chronic pain. But it's not wise to persevere through a task to completion *despite* the pain. No, that would be bad! In the context of chronic pain, grit can help you to adapt activities and exercise to make them doable, to seek rewarding social connections, or to pursue meaningful values and goals. You can use grit to lead a life more active, social, fulfilling, and fun. One of the few studies on grit in people with chronic pain found that older adults with low back pain and lots of grit were more likely to engage in self-directed exercise in comparison to people with less grit.[78] Self-directed exercise, meaning activity you choose to do on your own terms, forms a critical part of almost all beneficial pain management programs.

So how can you get grittier? Studies are trying to answer that exact question, but for now it seems that having a growth mindset represents an important piece of the puzzle. As we saw in the chapter on trauma and chronic pain, Carol Dweck proposed that some individuals have a growth mindset, meaning they believe that talent isn't fixed but rather something that dedication and hard work can cultivate. People with a growth mindset see failure as a sign of trying and reaching the edge of their abilities, not weakness or inadequacy. In that light, failure can work as a powerful instrument for success if you learn from it and apply its lessons to future endeavors.

Thanks to Gratitude

Gratitude is having a heyday—in the media, workplace, and schools—but being grateful has served as a cornerstone of spiritual practice and society more broadly for thousands of years. Remember, the real point of *Thanks-giving* isn't turkey and pumpkin pie.

We can appreciate the necessities of life, such as safe housing, enough food to eat, and clean water to drink, and we can be grateful for possessions, especially those that have emotional importance, including the family china or a baseball cap from childhood. Less tangible matters, such as family, friendships, and the ability to do what you love, can spark intense feelings of gratitude. Spiritual experiences—watching a dramatic sunset or feeling connected to something greater than yourself—also can yield intense feelings of appreciation.

Researchers who have studied gratitude found that it ties strongly to emotional, psychological, and social well-being. Several studies have shown that gratitude practices such as keeping a gratitude journal can help improve general well-being and happiness, but a recent meta-analysis suggests that a stand-alone gratitude exercise likely isn't enough to improve most health outcomes.[79] That said, combining a gratitude activity with standard medical and psychological care could offer a more effective solution.

Other researchers have determined that feeling grateful correlates with better sleep (best evidence), as well as healthier eating, better blood pressure, and improved blood-sugar control. In the lab of Andrew Steptoe at University College London, Marta Jackowska led a study that gave booklets to 119 women randomly assigned to write about either gratitude or everyday events for two weeks.[80] Along the way, the women received encouraging emails. Those randomized to the no-treatment control group received instructions to go about their normal lives and that they would do a writing assignment after three weeks. The study found that the gratitude writers reported increases in happiness, optimism, and quality of sleep; the greater the improvement in well-being, the greater the improvement in sleep quality and blood pressure reduction. This study helps us understand how something as simple as a gratitude activity can affect cardiovascular health; it might do so by decreasing blood pressure.

With pain specifically, gratitude practices typically form part of a larger collection of skills to develop. For example, I served as a co-investigator on a study led by Mary Janevic, another FIERCE mentee, at the School of Public Health at the University of Michigan. We evaluated a community health worker–led pain self-management program that combined positive activities including a gratitude practice and performing acts of kindness with traditional pain self-management training.[81] We mostly studied older African American adults living in Detroit and found that this approach resulted in decreased pain severity and greater improvement in pain-related functioning and pain self-efficacy. More than 85 percent of participants reported "better" or "much better" global functioning compared to the control group, in which only 25 percent reported similar improvement. That difference is huge and strongly supports the approach to pain self-management that we'll explore in the second part of this book: combining traditional pain-management skills with those that enhance positive emotions and well-being.

Grace and the Ripple Effect of Kindness

In the context of this chapter, grace refers to kindness and the healing power of doing kind acts for others as well as yourself. My favorite bumper sticker reads: "Practice random acts of kindness and senseless beauty." A lovely thought, but did you know that those altruistic acts have potentially powerful health effects associated with them? Even more than that, you, the orchestrator of the act, may have the most to gain. Studies have shown that the person doing the kind act tends to benefit more than the recipient of the kind act! Furthermore, kindness engenders more kindness; the recipient of the kind act, touched by the beauty of it, often decides to perform a kind act for someone else and so on.

Numerous studies show how powerful these acts of kindness can be for emotional and physical health. Conducting kind acts correlates with less depression, greater happiness, and better overall well-being, as a meta-analysis published by Lee Rowland and Oliver Scott Curry at the University of Oxford showed.[82] They also conducted an experiment to determine whether the nature of the acts impacted happiness differently. They tasked study participants with seven days of kindness activities to see whether it made a difference if the acts benefited strangers, friends, or the participants themselves (self-kindness). The experiment found that a strong relationship exists between the number of acts and the level of happiness. The greater the number, the happier the person. It also determined—a surprise!—that people were similarly happy if they performed their acts of kindness for friends, strangers, or themselves. Just being kind, in and of itself, seems to make people happier.

Volunteer Work

As one well-studied form of kindness, volunteering can function like powerful medicine for body, mind, and spirit. An interesting study explored data gathered from the Survey of Texas Adults. As with other studies, researchers found powerful benefits for volunteering, including improvements in mental and physical health, life satisfaction, social well-being, and

depression.[83] They also observed a cumulative effect, meaning that participating in several volunteer activities had an association with even greater
health benefits.

This same study was one of the first to explore two different types
of volunteer work: other-oriented and self-oriented. Other-oriented volunteering refers primarily to helping other people with activities related
to health, education, religion, human services, and youth development.
In contrast, examples of self-oriented volunteering include arts or culture, environmental protection, animal welfare, work-related service, or a
political campaign. The study found both forms of volunteer work beneficial, but the strongest effects between the two types looked different.
For other-oriented volunteering, the strongest benefit for the volunteer
applied to social well-being, while the strongest effect for the self-oriented
volunteer was on physical health. In other words, doing kind activities that
also feed your needs and interests might be most beneficial to your health!

Few studies have looked at how positive service affects people with
chronic pain specifically. But one study led by Elizabeth Salt at the University of Kentucky found that middle-aged women with chronic pain who
engaged in more volunteer activities reported less pain, a greater sense of
purpose in life, fewer depressive symptoms, and higher levels of physical
activity compared to those who volunteered less often.[84]

Self-Compassion

In the early part of my career, I noticed a striking pattern. Almost all my
patients described the habit of caring for others while neglecting themselves. Putting others first seemed remarkably brave and kind, but in the
long run it became unsustainable. Invariably, these patients felt burned out,
unappreciated, resentful, hurt, and often all the above. In this frazzled state,
they eventually couldn't fulfill the valued role of care provider, which dealt
a cruel blow to their self-esteem. You can see where this is going. Their pain
worsened as did their depression. So what's the answer? Self-compassion,
self-kindness, and self-care.

Self-compassion means giving yourself the same support, good advice, and leeway that you would give a friend or family member whom you like and respect. It's that simple. When you make a mistake, don't judge yourself more harshly than you would a dear friend. When you need support, don't tell yourself that you're weak and needy. You would never say that to someone you care about. Instead, give yourself permission to seek support. When you run out of energy and simply can't do any more, think about what you would say to a close friend in that situation. You might tell them to rest, do something pleasant, sleep—whatever it is, do that for yourself.

What's remarkable is that self-compassion is good for you. A recent meta-analysis examining more than ninety studies of self-compassion found that it predicts good outcomes for many health domains, with the strongest effects for overall physical health, positive health behaviors, sleep, and functional immunity.[85] Yes, you read that right, self-compassion can affect your immune system.

The bottom line: Learn how to be a better friend to yourself. Loving-kindness meditation, a powerful evidence-based activity, can help you improve your self-compassion and enhance positive emotions.[86] Listen to a recording at AftonHassett.com (Resources). Go on, give it a try.

Random Kindness, Senseless Beauty

Spreading kindness doesn't require lots of planning, and it can entail small acts such as paying someone a heartfelt compliment, holding the door for a stranger, or spending some extra time with a friend in need of company. More elaborate planning might have even greater benefits, though. The most effective approach appears to be planning and executing five acts of kindness all in one day. Planning and preparation make the acts more memorable, and the sustained period of anticipation and excitement likely boosts the emotional and physical benefits of the kind acts.

I hope I've convinced you that inviting more grit, gratitude, and grace into your life can help you harness your own natural healing powers. The second part of the book will give you some great activities for this purpose, but if you'd like to get a jump start, put this book down and do something kind for a stranger, something kind for someone you care about, and something kind for yourself.

IDEAS TO REMEMBER

- Grit means the long-term passion for and perseverance toward goals that help you achieve success on your terms.
- Gratitude is your heartfelt appreciation for worldly things as well as less tangible entities, such as family, friendships, and doing what you love. It also can be spiritual.
- Grace, in this context, refers to performing acts of kindness for others and yourself. Even small kind acts can have a beautiful ripple effect in the world.
- Practicing grit, gratitude, and grace has powerful benefits for your mental and physical health.
- Self-compassion—which means giving yourself the same understanding, patience, good advice, and love that you would give to a close friend—can improve your life and your experience of pain.

Lived Experience: Monica

I once believed that the sole purpose of pain was to act as a voice for the body when distressed, to protect it from further harm. However, my understanding about the purpose of pain forever changed about five years ago, when I became a person with chronic pain.

In 2018, I was a passenger in a catastrophic bus accident. I sustained devastating injuries to my neck, lumbar spine, and brain, along with many other painful wounds. These life-altering injuries upended my previously pleasant quality of life. To add insult to injury, the accident stole from me my beloved career as a licensed clinical social worker. Ouch! Three decades of social work–related service and building relationships with my clients gone in less than one minute.

My once-charmed life suddenly was replaced with a life consisting of surgical procedures, taking four different controlled substances, using adaptive devices, daily medical appointments, being monitored by *fifteen* different physician specialists, and relegation to nonemergency medical transportation in the form of multi-passenger vans.

Truly, this situation was more than surreal. It was soul-crushing to the extent that I was hoping for fewer days to live this new life, a life that seemed devoid of passion, pleasure, and purpose. I felt as though I had lost my reason for living. These recurring thoughts of loss and emptiness were my companions on my daily rides to and from appointments. Yet during these rides, I began to have a spiritual experience, and a new self-awareness emerged.

While being transported to and from medical appointments or sitting in lobby waiting rooms, strangers shared their life stories with me, and I learned about their paths to and their experiences of living with chronic pain. As I became aware of their various plights, I prayed for and with them. The more I prayed, the less attention I paid to the constant pain agonizing me twenty-four hours a day, and the more I experienced a greater understanding of the other purpose or purposes of pain.

Pain can aid or even accelerate the evolution of spiritual development.

Such spiritual development can result in greater spiritual faith, strength, courage, and wisdom to help withstand pain in the body and mind until it is removed or becomes more manageable. Through prayer—for me, that's talking to God—and in service to one another, an intimacy with something greater than ourselves is established, allowing us to witness the manifestation of answered prayer more frequently.

It's especially tempting to doubt the existence of God or His love for us in the event of prolonged bodily or emotional pain. If He existed, why is the pain not yet removed, or why don't other difficulties in life change as quickly as you believe they should?

Although I continue to suffer pain and discomfort, it's nowhere near the level it was at the start of this difficult journey. God has used an array of interventions that have passed through the heads, hands, and hearts of medical professionals and scientists, coupled with my dedication to prayer to transform me from a social worker to *soul*-cial worker. In 2019, I became an ordained minister with the Universal Life Church. My life now has great purpose and meaning despite the pain. I hope the same will be true for you.

Be well. I'll be praying for you.

———

Monica Gay is an ordained minister and soul-cial worker.

14

IN AWE OF SOMETHING GREATER

Awe singularly evokes both the notion that we are small but also that we are significant in a universe where something much bigger and infinitely more magnificent exists.

The Science of Awe

Before 2000, little research in this area existed but since then investigators have shown increasing interest in understanding what the experience of awe means to mind and body. Think of awe as a state or emotion that evokes a relatively predictable series of thoughts and feelings. Now ponder this question. Can a white paper really be inspirational?

Yes! The Greater Good Science Center at the University of California at Berkeley prepared just such a white paper for the John Templeton Foundation in 2018.[87] In it, Summer Allen beautifully summarized the current science regarding awe. She noted that "awe is often accompanied by feelings of self-diminishment and increased connectedness with other people. Experiencing awe often puts people in a self-transcendent state where they focus less on themselves and feel more like a part of a larger whole. In this way, awe can be considered an altered state of consciousness, akin to a flow state, in addition to an emotional state."

The white paper proposes that many types of stimuli can evoke a feeling of awe, including but not limited to: spiritual practices, nature, visual and performing arts, grand architecture, and acts of kindness, bravery, and love. Awe evolved in humans perhaps because it can benefit survival by enhancing social connections through powerful shared experience, forcing us to take in and adapt to new information (increasing our cognitive flexibility) and appreciating vast spaces that could contain threats or treats—from a safe distance of course.

Whatever the source or evolutionary benefit, awe seems to have health benefits. First, it can make us feel happier, less stressed, more humble, less depressed, and more caring, with greater life satisfaction. Awe provokes *reliable* physiological reactions, often including goosebumps or chills (sometimes called "goose-tingles"), and has other physiological effects such as healthy activation of the autonomic nervous system and changes to the immune system that may help decrease the harmful effects of stress and inflammation.

To better understand how the brain processes awe, Ryota Takano and Michio Nomura at Kyoto University in Japan conducted a fascinating study in which people watched awe-inspiring videos while undergoing brain scans.[88] The researchers found that positive awe experiences activated neural networks involved in aesthetic reward processing (*Oh, so beautiful*) as well as those that process how we think about ourselves in connection to others. (*We are one.*) As we have learned, experiences that activate reward-processing areas of the brain might be particularly important for people with chronic pain. So where should we go and what should we do to get some awe?

Nature and Awe

Nature generates powerful feelings of awe because of its vastness and power. Large outdoor spaces often evoke it. Picture a purple mountain range stretching across the landscape, the Grand Canyon, miles of golden grass blowing rhythmically across rolling plains, thousands of stars scattered across the night sky, or the ocean crashing on jagged rocks. Impossibly big and incomparably beautiful spaces can imply something greater at work. How else could something so astounding exist?

In a study conducted by Matthew Ballew and Allen Omoto at the Claremont Graduate University in California, they randomly assigned 100 people to sit either in a natural environment, such as an arboretum, or a built outdoor environment, like a sports stadium.[89] Participants remained in their respective locations for fifteen minutes with instructions to focus on their surroundings. Next, they rated their feelings. Investigators found that the participants in the natural setting reported significantly greater feelings of awe and other positive emotions, including happiness and contentment, compared to those seated in a man-made structure. Feeling captivated by or engrossed in the environment seemed to explain the powerful impact that nature had on these positive emotions.

But not all awe is peaceful or pleasant, which explains the difference between the words "awesome" and "awful." Devastating forest fires, swollen rivers flooding, and hurricane-force winds showcase the brutality of nature and can evoke reverence (awe) for events that render us small and vulnerable. While not joyful, this kind of awe still causes us to ponder our place in the universe and bonds us to others in a way that could promote survival.

When the forces of nature aren't threatening to engulf us, nature is great for us. Even city dwellers have an innate need to get outside among greenery and water, which has given rise to nature therapy and shinrin-yoku, the traditional Japanese practice of "forest bathing." These practices involve immersing yourself in nature in a mindful way that engages all the senses, and studies have found that intentionally spending time in this way can inspire awe and has positive effects on mental health, attention and focus, heart rate and blood pressure, and the immune system.[90] A study from Japan evaluating the practice of forest bathing showed a 50 percent increase in the number of natural killer cells—a critical component of your immune system—after people completed a three-day retreat.[91] Elevation in these powerful disease-fighting cells lasted for as long as two weeks *after* the retreat. If a pill offered that kind of effect, some pharmaceutical company would have a new best-seller!

Outdoor spaces closer to home can have health benefits, too. A simple walk in the park or spending time in your yard or garden can have positive health effects. The healing power of gardens, which falls under the canopy of horticultural therapy, can result in improvements in stress, depression, and anxiety.[92] Flowers delight multiple senses, and cultivating fresh fruit and vegetables can contribute to healthier eating. So regular exposure to natural spaces can make us healthier and happier. The key is not just to spend time in these spaces but to do so like a child, taking in everything—sights, sounds, smells, textures, and tastes—with openness and wonder.

The Arts and Awe

Have you ever been listening to music and suddenly felt involuntarily chills when the piece hits a crescendo or the music touches on something tender or meaningful? Those chills might differ slightly from awe. Awe includes the sense of self-diminishment, or feeling small in a good way, while also feeling connected to others. The arts certainly can inspire awe, but that means more than just the chills. We're talking those full-on, full-body tingles that for me was the first time I heard Beethoven's Ninth Symphony in a concert hall (a shared experience) with the clearly delineated crescendo that practically screams, *Clutch your armrests and get ready for some serious* awe!

Music has some remarkable health benefits. Studies in dementia show that musical memories have a surprising resistance to deterioration. They also demonstrate how music therapy can improve cognitive function, depression, and quality of life in people with dementia.[93] Quite a few studies have explored the value of music for reducing the experience of pain in people with acute and chronic pain. Music decreases acute pain related to surgery and childbirth, while for chronic pain, it can reduce pain severity, improve mood, and decrease anxiety.[94] A key element of the effectiveness of these studies was the type and likeability of the music. Music has a greater positive effect when people choose their own music.

A particularly moving drama can inspire awe, as can a musical that culminates in a powerful synchronous dance number. Think of "One Singular Sensation" from *A Chorus Line* or the dark but electric "Cell Block Tango" from *Chicago*. Visual arts can be moving as well. Every year, more than six million people wait in long lines to see the enigmatic smile of the Mona Lisa, another six million visit the Sistine Chapel to stare up at that remarkable ceiling, and over eight million flock to see the splendor of the Taj Mahal. We crave awe, we want to be impressed by grandeur, beauty, and accomplishment.

Bringing more beauty into your life has documented health benefits. In a series of studies led by Tores Theorell at the Karolinska Institute in Stockholm, his team found a range of benefits associated with different art experiences.[95] For example, a group of older women viewed and discussed various works of art and, compared to control groups, reported feeling happier and less depressed and having healthier blood pressure. In another study, people with IBS either sang in a choir once a week for six months or didn't (the control group). The choir singers experienced less inflammation and showed a trend toward experiencing less pain. In a third study, people with fibromyalgia either took part in a weekly dance class or received their usual care for a six-month period. The study found that the dance class participants had less pain, greater mobility, and more energy. These studies and many others demonstrate just some of the powerful healing effects of the arts.

Cue the Music

Her face bathed in soft blue light, she stared at the leafy and starry ceiling. Stone columns carved to resemble trees branching outward to form a geometric canopy towered above at dizzying heights. Light cascading down from stained glass windows enveloped the interior space of the Sagrada Familia Cathedral in a riot of greens, blues, yellows, and reds. The vibrant colors sparkled and danced, infusing life into the gray stone, and touching the souls of the humans made small by the majesty of the building. It was our mother-daughter trip to Europe. My mother had never crossed the

Atlantic before to see the great cities she knew from books or dark movie theaters as an inquisitive little girl. We had explored Paris, Florence, Venice, Rome, and now Barcelona, cherishing our days strolling together through landmarks and museums and gratefully enjoying long lunches at sidewalk cafés. As we stood staring at the gigantic pipe organ barreling up the wall of the cathedral, her eyes welled with tears. *"It's just so beautiful,"* she whispered, then a minute later: "If only that pipe organ would play, then it would be perfect."

As if heard by an angel, the space suddenly filled with sublime music gently breaking the din of hushed murmurs. We looked at each other with wide eyes and astonished smiles. Chills surged through our bodies, as an incomparable feeling overcame us. Sharing that powerful moment of awe drew us even closer together.

Selfless Acts of Love and Beauty

Sometimes we surprise one another. An ordinary person can act in an extraordinary way by showing incredible selflessness, bravery, or altruism. In our recent discussion of kindness, we noted that both the performer of a kind act and the recipient can reap psychological and potentially physiological benefits. Altruism can have powerful health benefits that might be more pronounced in women. In a study of people with painful lumbar spine disorders, participants reported similar levels of altruism, but for women higher levels of altruism had greater health benefits, including less pain.[96]

Spirituality and Awe

For spiritual people, awe can manifest most consistently during spiritual practice, whether at religious services, while praying or meditating, or during a quiet nature walk. The Pew Foundation long has surveyed global trends in religious affiliation, noting that roughly 85 percent of people have a religious affiliation, a number that may be growing.[97] Furthermore, most people without a formal religious affiliation still believe in a higher power, considering themselves spiritual people.

Spirituality denotes the sense of connection to something greater than ourselves. Aligning with the definition of awe, it often includes the strong sense of being connected to other people in a deep and meaningful way. Spiritual practice can be a solo endeavor, but frequently it involves activities that bring people together to worship and commune. Such fellowship might be a key element of the mental and physical health benefits of spiritual practice. Studies that explore the mental and physical health benefits of spirituality indicate that spirituality correlates with less depression, lower rates of substance abuse, and less suicidality and may promote improved health outcomes (fewer heart attacks and strokes), better family functioning, greater life satisfaction, and lower mortality.[98]

A few studies have explored the associations between spirituality and the experience of pain in chronic pain populations. For example, a recent study found that, when people with pain viewed spirituality as providing hope and a positive perspective toward life, that perspective had an association with better psychological function and coping responses.[99] Those individuals could ignore pain and use coping self-statements more effectively. Further, when spirituality supported the search for meaning and purpose in life, it correlated with coping using task persistence. When couched in terms of support and living a purposeful life, spirituality seems to offer an excellent route by which pain exerts less power on day-to-day living.

In Search of Awe

Putting yourself in awe-inspiring situations can be a fun and beneficial endeavor. If we stay in our homes, holed up in our beds, not experiencing the remarkable places, people, or events in the world, we miss an opportunity to grow and add (more) meaning to our lives. One of the activities you'll try during the thirty-day program will be planning an "aweliday." It's my way of nudging you toward some awe-inspired goose-tingles.

IDEAS TO REMEMBER

- Awe involves feeling positive self-diminishment and an increased connectedness with other people. In feeling awe, people focus less on themselves and feel more like part of a larger whole.
- Nature, artistic expression, architectural achievements, exceptional human acts, and spiritual practices all can spark awe, to name just a few.
- Positive-awe experiences activate brain networks involved in reward processing and other neural networks that process how we think about ourselves in connection with others. Those experiences and activating those brain networks are particularly important for people with chronic pain.
- Experiencing awe-inspiring situations, such as visiting interesting places or seeing amazing objects, is good for you on many levels! Go on, seek some awe.

Lived Experience: Kathleen

After chronic pain made itself at home in my body, I felt defeated. I had been active and vital but then had to accept that I likely would never travel again and not even get out much. Throughout the winter months, I essentially became homebound. While I wasn't suicidal, I felt that, at age fifty-two, I was ready to go. The best of life lay behind me. Moving forward, I just would be biding time, enduring, and then at some point blessedly fading away. In this dark time, I often wondered, *Why am I here?* I felt this way most poignantly when hearing of a child or young person passing. Why couldn't God or the universe spare them and take me instead?

But then I started noticing things that were meaningful or lovely, and I was glad I was here. If I died when I felt so ready to go, I would've missed these experiences. I also started noticing how I was still helpful to others, though I felt that I had lost most of the usefulness in my quiet, simple life. With those frustrated by COVID restrictions, I had unique wisdom and insights to share because I'd been adjusting to isolation and restriction for many years prior. When a friend said that my advice helped him through a rough patch at work, I thought, *Maybe this is why I'm still here. Maybe I've been languishing these past few years just to reach this point of helping one friend.*

With this new perspective, I began to see other reasons that I might be here. For example, I am the only one who can give our cat his daily medication. What if an essential part of the greater plan is that I keep this magical creature healthy and thriving? That would be enough. Maybe it's about others rather than me. I continued to pay attention: my husband's love, lively conversations with friends, the pleasure in cooking and eating a great meal. Perhaps this is why I've lasted this long.

No matter how insignificant my actions and experiences may seem, I've come to believe them essential to the universal tapestry. Each is a thread integral to the whole. I am needed. I used to believe that a life without physical comfort and ability, with the freedom to engage in life's array of offerings was less-than, something to be regretted and endured. Now I know that, if I learn something, share my love, or help someone each day, then it's been a wonderful day. The bug I rescued and released outside this morning may be the reason I woke today. The prayers for healing and peace that I send to others might be finding their mark.

As I've honed my attention, serendipity often amazes me, which further assures me that I'm precisely where I'm supposed to be. This present creation, this moment's arising humble me. I cannot be certain of the specific reasons that I'm here, why each occurrence arises, but I can marvel at the possibilities, and I can be certain that I'm needed here, in this life. When I'm needed elsewhere, I'll be elsewhere. I no longer wish for the end or wonder why I continue to live. I'm here to love, learn, and receive all the light, shadow, joy, and sorrow that each moment delivers in abundance. *This* is why I'm here.

———

Kathleen Sutherland is a writer, creative baker, and spiritual explorer.

15

PURPOSE IN LIFE AND
THE WAY FORWARD

Kathleen's story captures a common experience that many people with chronic pain have when their vision for their life, goals, hopes, and aspirations completely derails. In this disruption, your senses of self and purpose can get lost. Our roles often dictate how we see ourselves—professional, partner, parent, friend, artist, or athlete—but not being able to fulfill these roles in ways we judge adequate can leave us feeling lost. Efforts to make the pain go away can feel all-consuming and pursued at the expense of fulfilling these roles. It becomes a conundrum. This loss of self and meaning sets the stage for helplessness and hopelessness. Depression and insidious thoughts of doom creep in. It's human and normal to have these thoughts or feelings for a moment or two but give yourself permission to dismiss them. If you can't stop thinking these thoughts or shake the weight of depression, seek professional care. This book isn't enough. Flip to the Resources section on page 255 to start seeking direct, professional help.

So how can we balance what we *can* do with what we *want* to do? How can we lead a life that feels more rewarding and meaningful despite the pain? Let's look at why we need to focus on building a more purposeful life.

The Power of Purpose

Studies evaluating the benefits of having a strong sense of purpose in life have shown that it correlates with better sleep, better diet and nutrition, improved immune function, and healthier aging, including preventative health behaviors such as getting a colonoscopy, cholesterol test, or mammogram. Other studies show that purpose in life has an association with better health outcomes: reduced risk for heart attacks, decreased incidence of stroke, decreased risk for Alzheimer's disease, improved diabetes, and less depression and anxiety. For people with chronic pain, a couple of studies look especially pertinent.

In a study led by Eric Kim at the Harvard T. H. Chan School of Public Health, our team at the University of Michigan, including purpose-in-life expert Vic Strecher—as well as well-being luminary Carol Ryff from the University of Wisconsin—explored the possibility that a strong sense of purpose in life could decrease the risk for misuse of prescription drugs.[100] As you can imagine, this topic remains a critical area in pain research and clinical care in the context of the opioid epidemic and the common misuse of other substances (prescription drugs, alcohol, even street drugs) to self-manage pain, emotional or physical. We evaluated 3,535 middle-aged adults from the Midlife in the United States Study who weren't misusing drugs when first surveyed to see how they were doing nine to ten years later. We compared people with the highest levels of purpose to those with the lowest levels and found that a strong sense of purpose greatly decreased the odds of future drug misuse even when taking into consideration other common risk factors such as psychological distress, the presence of other diseases and conditions, and health behaviors including smoking and alcohol consumption.

A different study that also used data from the Midlife in the United States Study database explored the relationship between purpose in life and chronic pain. The goal was to use a more nuanced approach to understand what it is to lead a life filled with meaning. Led by Brandon Boring, the team at Texas A&M University proposed that the complex idea of living a meaningful life involves three distinct facets: knowing your life purpose; mattering or feeling like your life matters to yourself and others; and your life having coherence. That third idea might need a little explanation. Coherence means that your life makes sense. Think of the common phrase: "Everything happens for a reason." A sense of coherence implies an overarching order to life.

To explore the role of each of these facets—purpose, mattering, and coherence—in chronic pain, the investigators conducted three studies.[101] First, they explored the relationships among the three facets and the development of chronic pain nine years later. In the second study, they explored associations between the three facets and pain severity in young adults. Then, in the third study, they tracked changes in pain severity over four weeks and mapped fluctuations in severity onto the three facets. In the first study, they found that having a strong sense of coherence uniquely correlated with fewer headaches and less pain in the back, joints, and extremities (arms, hands, legs, feet). More importantly, having a strong sense of coherence reduced the odds of developing chronic pain over the nine-year timespan. Coherence also had an association with decreased pain severity (second study) and best predicted fluctuations in weekly pain severity (third study). Unexpectedly, the concept of "mattering" was associated with more frequent back pain in the first study and greater pain severity in the second study. Boring and his colleagues speculated that a sense of mattering can involve focusing on how your life impacts others or has greater meaning. Chronic pain imposing limitations that thwart these expectations could result in stress at not being able to fulfill that role. Whatever stresses you out likely worsens your pain.

Mortality, or whether someone lives or dies, might offer one of the most compelling outcomes. A meta-analysis evaluating studies that tracked more than 130,000 people over time addressed the question of whether people with a strong sense of purpose in life live longer.[102] Even when considering critical health factors—including age, general health, and having heart disease—investigators still found that purpose in life was associated with a 17 percent reduction in the risk of death. If you heard about a medication that powerful, wouldn't you consider taking it?

Purpose in Life and Pain: A Caveat

A note of caution for people with chronic pain. The study conducted by Brandon Boring and the team at Texas A&M revealed some counterintuitive findings regarding purpose in life and the development or worsening of pain. For some people, purpose in life might have made their pain worse. The researchers speculated that—because pain interferes with the ability to meet life goals, thus derailing the fulfillment of purpose—stress, anxiety, and depression can result and make the pain worse or even chronic.

So your purpose in life needs to feel congruent with your limitations, whatever they might be. In other words, managing expectations is important. For us mere mortals, this psychological flexibility often takes place in adolescence or early adulthood, when, for example, the ambitions that dominate childhood (astronaut, athlete, president, rock star) yield to more realistic career goals. Societal constraints, educational opportunities, family finances, physical limitations, raw talent, and dumb luck all conspire to make many paths unrealistic, but that doesn't mean that the realistic way forward lacks purpose or meaning. Limitations, including pain, can't stop us from leading purposeful lives *if we so choose*. We only need to establish, not find, new purpose.

Establishing, Modifying, or Pursuing
Purpose in Life: A Primer

I hadn't thought much about the meaning of my life until about seven or eight years ago when teaching a class of freshmen at the University of Michigan. I've taught a first-year seminar called "Happiness and Health: The Science of Resilience," off and on, for almost a decade. An honor and a joy, it has been perhaps my most meaningful act as an academic and maybe as a human. The bright, young students learn about research methodology and how to search and consider the scientific literature. But they also try many of the same evidence-based activities that appear in Part Two of this book. They learn so much about themselves and one another while establishing skills that can help promote happiness throughout their lives.

A student once asked me: "Dr. Hassett, what's *your* purpose in life?"

A spark of panic may have flashed in my eyes because I had never put the answer into words. After a moment of reflection, I responded: "My purpose in life is to teach you all, and as many other people as possible, simple life skills that will help you lead happier and more rewarding lives."

Since that day, my purpose in life has felt clear. Knowing my purpose helps guide daily decisions about what I do and how I structure my time. This knowledge dictates the direction of my research and even inspired the writing of this book.

Where can you begin if your purpose doesn't feel clear? When you have chronic pain, your journey might require some extra psychological flexibility. Are you willing to let go of goals that aren't realistic or gratifying? Sometimes people choose paths that fulfill a desire of someone else, such as a parent or spouse. You should set your own purpose, which aligns with your values and feels personally meaningful. It's not out there somewhere, awaiting discovery like a rare coin or stamp; *you* establish your purpose in life based on your values, interests, abilities, and passions. Start thinking about it to give yourself a leg up for the exploration section later.

Through defining your own unique purpose in life, you not only will feel more at peace, but you also will also feel energized. Even on bad days, you still can wake up with a desire to seize the day. You might need to modify your activities to accommodate how you feel, but what you do can still align with your sense of purpose. Each day is precious. It's all we have, so carpe diem!

IDEAS TO REMEMBER

- People with a strong sense of purpose in life take better care of themselves and enjoy a decreased risk for heart attacks, stroke, Alzheimer's disease, depression, substance misuse, and chronic pain.

- A strong sense of coherence, or believing that life makes sense, may be particularly helpful for people with chronic pain.

- Role disruption can derail your sense of direction, meaning, and purpose. Charting a new way forward in the face of life's challenges may not feel easy, but it's worth it.

- You don't find your purpose in life; you *establish* it based on your values, interests, abilities, and passions.

PREPARING FOR YOUR JOURNEY

The practice of qigong typically includes the execution of a series of movements that promote the free flow of qi ("chee"), or energy, throughout the body to encourage good health. In a park, you might have seen people following a leader performing these graceful movements. In *external* qigong therapy, a qigong master uses his or her hands to apply intense pressure to specific points in the body, waves hands vigorously over the body, and performs cupping (applying a small, heated cup to the skin to create suction) to liberate blocked qi in another person.

Len Sigal, then chief of rheumatology at Robert Wood Johnson Medical School and one of my earliest mentors, introduced me to Kevin Chen and encouraged us to collaborate. Through Kevin's work in traditional Chinese medicine, he had met a qigong master who claimed that he was curing people with chronic pain using external qigong therapy. In science, when discussing the treatment of chronic pain, we seldom or never use the word "cure." We aim for meaningful improvement, but *cure*? No. I wanted to study the phenomenon if only to debunk a false claim. As a woman of science, I was—to put it kindly—skeptical.

On the first day of our study, Kevin and I met our study participants as a group and told the volunteers more about the study. They read and signed their consent forms, which noted, in part, that some of the activities could cause pain and even bruising. As if on cue, a young, fit, and vibrant man wearing a navy-blue tracksuit and running shoes burst into the room. Not at all what I imagined, he nonetheless took control declaring that he was ready to start and that the first participant should follow him into the exam room. His eyes flashed my way, and he said that I could observe if I liked. Yes, please.

A padded exam table stood in the middle of the too-small exam room, with a second pushed up against the wall. The research assistant was sitting on the second exam table, her back against the wall, clipboard in hand. I hopped up beside her.

The qigong therapy session began. The first volunteer—a quiet, middle-aged woman with a sweet sense of humor—lay on the exam table, stomach down, as instructed. Like all the participants for this study, she had a diagnosis of fibromyalgia with severe chronic pain throughout her body. The qigong master applied intense pressure to muscle tissue in her upper back. She screamed so loud that I almost screamed along with her! *What the hell is he doing?* I thought.

"Shall I continue?" the master asked.

"Yes, go ahead. I'm fine," she replied. Her response surprised me. I would have been less shocked had she leapt up and smacked him, but she didn't.

More pressure, more screaming, more requests to continue, more permission granted.

The room felt stiflingly hot, and I began to sweat. This was where my career was going to end. Security surely was going to burst into the room to see who was being assaulted and hold me accountable. As I wiped away the sweat, the qigong master turned to me.

"You are warm," he said. "We all feel it."

The research assistant glanced at me and nodded.

"Energy is moving," the master continued. "Come here and put your hands by her feet."

I obeyed and placed both hands about six inches from her feet, fingers up and palms toward her. He vigorously waved his hands a few inches over her body, making brushing motions like moving water in a shallow pool. He paused for a few seconds, hands over her body, eyes closed. He stood back, dropped his hands, and asked, "What do you feel now?"

A faint stream of cool air seemed to be flowing from her feet, like a gentle breeze. I couldn't explain it. I couldn't believe it. The master said that I was feeling the exchange of energy, warm for cool, and that the volunteer would feel better. Weeks later, after several painful treatments, she indeed felt much better.

All the scientific knowledge I have gained over the years still fails to account for what took place that day and the weeks that followed. I know only what our data told us. Quite a few volunteers showed robust improvement in pain, functioning, and depression. *The Journal of Alternative and Complementary Medicine* published the results of our pilot study in 2006.[103] Only much larger, randomized controlled trials can prove the potential effectiveness of this treatment, but to date, no such studies have taken place. Nonetheless, I learned once again that we simply don't understand so much about the brain, the body, and life, so it's best to remain open and curious. You never know when something extraordinary might happen.

Are You Ready?

I hope so! You kindly have given me the gift of your attention as we covered a vast array of subjects from neuroscience to spirituality. By now, I hope you understand or at least remain open to the notion that the brain lies at the center of the pain experience and that how you think, feel, and act can influence how your brain processes that pain signal: amplifying it, dampening it, ignoring it, or even conjuring it. We've discussed how stress, fear, resentment, hopelessness, anger, and sadness supercharge the brain's pain circuits and that choosing joy, friendship, calm, love, purpose, and fun ameliorates it. I encourage you to re-read the Ideas to Remember sections at the end of each chapter, which will refresh your memory about why seemingly unrelated things matter. I'll wait here while you do that, patiently listening to background music. ("The Girl from Ipanema," we'll go with that.)

**Re-read all the Ideas to Remember summaries
at the end of every chapter. Yes, now, please.**

Welcome Back!

So I bet that you're even more curious about trying the activities, practices, and skills I've been mentioning. Based on scientific evidence, these are designed to improve your pain and ability to function directly and indirectly. The daily activities appear in an intentional order based on the principles of cognitive-behavioral therapy, my experience in clinical practice and research, and the advice of my ridiculously smart colleagues who helped me plan this book.

First, you'll learn a few skills that you can use any time to calm your mind and decrease your physiological stress response. These centering skills not only can help you cope better with stress but also come in handy for improving your sleep, which is addressed next. Perhaps you've begun improving your sleep by experimenting with sleep-time stablization or trying some of the sleep-promoting practices we discussed in Chapter 8. Either way, you'll try changing other habits that can make good sleep elusive. After that, it's time to get more exercise: not boring, painful calisthenics from the 1940s, but fun exercise that takes you to cool places and encourages you to do interesting activities. Then comes a series of days to explore ways to better manage your thoughts and emotions. Throughout the process, you'll discover strategies to help you lead a life that feels more active, connected, rewarding, and fun. Much of what you will try builds *life* skills that can be beneficial for all people, with and without pain. Share them with others because, as you recall, acts of kindness are good for your health!

How It's Going to Work

Every day for the next thirty days, you'll try a different activity, practice, or skill based on scientific evidence. That means that research already has indicated that it's helpful for people with chronic medical conditions.

Read about it, think about it, then try it *that same day*. This next point is critical. Even if you've tried something before and know you like or dislike it, do it one more time in the context of this program. At the end of the day, go back to the activity page and take stock of how it went and whether you might want to add it to your Thriving Plan later. Each activity has a star that you can check, circle, or color to help you remember the keepers. Before you make that decision, think about the following critical idea.

One day of training won't allow you to run a marathon. In the same way, trying a new activity for one day isn't enough of a "dose" to experience instant pain improvement, immediately better sleep, or a suddenly joyous mood. One day of trying something won't make your pain or other symptoms disappear.

Still, you really need to *try the activity*. Your reset will work only if you remain active and committed, identifying and building the skills you need and like. To remind yourself to stay on track, put a sticky note on the refrigerator, add it to your calendar, or set a reminder on your smartphone. Place this book next to your alarm clock or beside your bed so you see it first thing in the morning and last thing at night. Come up with the best no-fail strategy to remind you of your committment to improving your life for the next thirty days and beyond. To stay accountable, consider taking this journey with a trusted friend or loved one and form a Chronic Pain Reset (CPR) team. Set a prize for completing the thirty-day period or for the team member(s) who have the biggest breakthrough. Do whatever works as long as you commit to spending at least fifteen minutes a day trying the activities.

FAQ

Here are some frequently asked questions and related answers, observations, and suggestions.

Where Do These Activities, Practices, and Skills Come From?

They are evidence-based and come from cognitive behavioral therapy (CBT) for pain and from second-generation, CBT-based approaches, such as mindfulness-based stress reduction (MBSR), acceptance and commitment therapy (ACT), positive psychotherapy, dialectical behavioral therapy (DBT), and emotion-focused CBT for pain (PRT, EAET, etc.).

What If an Activity Resonates Right Away and I Want to Keep Doing It?

Then, do it! The goal is to build your own Thriving Plan. If you find something that seems to work, stick with it. You might be an early starter, so go for it.

What If Something Sounds Stupid and Couldn't Possibly Be Helpful?

Here's where I call on you to be especially open and curious. Please give it a try anyway. We don't understand so much about the brain and body, and sometimes something just . . . *works*. Really, what do you have to lose? At worst, it'll make you laugh or become fodder for a good story later.

What If I Like Too Many of the Activities?

Ha! This would be a great problem. Even if you have starred twenty-five of the thirty activities, that's fine. Remember that you will not be doing all of them all at once, now or later. When you build your Thriving Plan later in this book, you will prioritize amongst the activities you like and need most and just do one or two at a time. Other activities will be added later.

What Are Domains?

For each day's activity, you might notice "Domains" with a list of treatment domains such as Physical Activity, Better Sleep, or Positive Emotion. It's not necessary to take treatment domains into consideration now, but these will be important when you build your Thriving Plan.

What If I'm Having an Awful Day and Simply Can't?

Here, you have options. Read the day's activity and see if it sounds doable. If not, take a day off and try the activity the next day. If you're doing the challenge with others, read about it, discuss it with your CPR team, and/or ask them to take a breather with you. The journey will take thirty-one days, and that's OK. After all, it's *your* journey.

Do You Have Any Tips or Tricks?

I do. First, you already have what you need to succeed. Reading this book shows that you have the *desire*. You have acquired so much *knowledge* that can help you understand why these activities, practices, and skills can help. You also have your character *strengths* to get you through the tough parts. Lean on those strengths, values, and vision for your more rewarding life when circumstances, people, or that old, unhelpful thinking tries to lure you away.

———

One more time, the big question: *Are you ready?* If so, let's go!

Lived Experience: Michele

My mother is one of ten children—yes, *ten*. Raised in rural Jamaica, in a culture steeped in patriarchy, she was baptized in the waters of self-denial. Starting at age seven, she and my grandmother woke at 5:00 a.m. to make breakfast for her dad and seven brothers. When the men left, she made their beds and prepared her brothers' clothes for when they returned at 8:00 a.m. to get ready for school. In the evening, my mom helped her mother prepare and serve dinner and clean up after the men before doing her homework. Putting others before herself was embedded in her DNA.

As a child, I remembered Mom seeming to be in multiple places at once. She was a teacher and a caretaker who was always available for me and my siblings, the countless cousins who lived with us over the years, her students, and the kids from our church. Yet I never remembered her taking time for herself. She always accepted interruption to whatever she was doing because I needed something. My siblings remember the same thing. The many people who relied on her were always her priority.

Today, my ninety-three-year-old mom is still my hero and my model for motherhood. I also inherited her tendency for self-denial. When an autoimmune disease resulted in chronic pain, I continued my life as a mother and caregiver without making plans to do anything differently. I guess subconsciously my self-denial default honored the legacy and sacrifice of my mother. If she did it, then so should I. I wore my Strong Black Woman superhero cape with pride. I accepted my struggle with pain as just something that is.

One day, I was in the kitchen making tea for Mom and me when my younger daughter called my mobile. I put her on speaker and she asked me to take her and two friends to a local theme park on Saturday. I told her that I needed to cancel a physical therapy appointment that day, but I'd be happy to do it.

"Mom, it's OK," she said. "We can go another day."

I insisted that it wasn't a problem.

After the call, my mom was giving me a disapproving look. She asked why I didn't accept my daughter's offer to reschedule their plans. It never occurred to me to consider my needs above those of my daughter, even though I had been in pain for several days and didn't know how quickly I could book another PT appointment. That observation, coming from my mom of all people, forced me to examine the quality of the relationship I had with myself and whether I thought that I ever deserved to put myself first. If my joints could talk, how would they describe my care for them? How about my emotional needs or need for sleep?

As mothers, daughters, friends, romantic partners, and workers, so many women living with chronic pain operate on automatic pilot, prioritizing everyone except themselves. You wouldn't think I'd have to say this, but I do. Your pain is important. You are important. So I challenge you today to begin a new chapter in your life. This might be one of the most important chapters, perhaps even a turning point. Let's start today and call it: "Priority: Me."

———

Michele Andwele is a public health professional; diversity, equity, and inclusion specialist; and social justice advocate.

PART TWO

Thirty Activities, Practices, and Skills for a Better Life

PACED BREATHING

DOMAINS: RELAXATION, BETTER SLEEP

How you breathe is a superpower. Paul Lehrer, one of my earliest mentors, instrumentally developed and tested this technique that teaches ordinary people how to shift the functioning of their autonomic nervous system subtly. The method decreases revving sympathetic activity and increases calming parasympathetic activity. Remember the sympathetic nervous system is what cues your fight-flight-or-freeze response. All you have to do is slow your breathing by decreasing the number of breaths you take per minute, inhaling slowly through your nose in a way that extends your abdomen and exhaling through pursed lips.

The breathing practices of yogis—masters of controlling automatic bodily processes that typically lie beyond our ability to influence, such as blood pressure—inspired this technique. Lehrer studied yogis in the Himalayas, who, when meditating, take about six breaths per minute and appear to exist in a relaxed and peaceful state.

Many studies have shown that paced breathing can help both pain and depression with an endless array of benefits for body and mind, including improving brain activity related to emotional control and psychological well-being. Ready to check it out?

Try It Today

- In a quiet place where you won't be disturbed, either lie down or sit comfortably in a chair with your feet flat on the floor.
- Place one hand on your upper chest and the other hand just below your rib cage.
- Slowly breathe in through your nose deeply enough so you feel your stomach rise while the hand on your chest stays as still as possible. As you inhale slowly count to five.
- Exhale, feeling your stomach fall inward under your hand as you exhale through pursed lips, as you would blow out birthday candles. Again, count slowly to five.
- Repeat these slow breath cycles for five minutes.
- As you practice your breathing, you can direct your attention to your breath, something in the room, or a breathing pacer. When your mind wanders, gently bring it back to whatever you have chosen for your focus point.
- Note how you feel afterward.

To aid your practice, you can find a breathing pacer at AftonHassett.com (Resources).

Make It Part of Your Thriving Plan

Throughout the day, take a couple of breaks to pace your breathing. This powerful technique can come in handy if you feel stressed, angry, or anxious. It helps your parasympathetic nervous system quiet feelings of fight, flight, or freeze. If you like this technique and want to make it a central part of your plan, practice it for twenty minutes or more per day to make it the most effective. Feel free to break that time into shorter segments if you like. The more you practice this technique, the better the physiological results.

PROGRESSIVE MUSCLE RELAXATION

DOMAINS: RELAXATION, BETTER SLEEP

Life leads to lots of stress, and for people with chronic pain, stress tends to make pain worse, particularly through muscle tension. We often tense our muscles without even realizing it, especially in the neck, shoulders, and lower back. Some people tense their fists, others clench their jaw muscles. Think about where you carry your stress so you can begin to release it.

A great counterintuitive way to control muscle tension is to tense your muscles. A technique called progressive muscle relaxation (PMR) prompts you to tense your muscles and then release that tension. You tighten and relax muscle groups in your body, one by one, starting with your toes and working upward to your face. Because we often don't realize that we're tightening our muscles, PMR helps bring awareness to how tension feels and gives you the power to relax. As with any skill, it works best if you practice it regularly. Like exercise, the more you do it, the better the results; and if you stop practicing, the results can start to fade.

Studies show that PMR can help a wide range of diseases and conditions, including chronic pain, high blood pressure, sleep problems, migraines, and anxiety.

Try It Today

- In a quiet place where you won't be disturbed for about fifteen minutes, sit or lie down comfortably.
- Take a deep breath as you tense each muscle group, in the order noted below.
- Hold your breath and the muscle tension for five seconds.
- Exhale as you release the tension.
- Rest for ten to twenty seconds, breathing comfortably, before moving to the next muscle group.

It's that easy! For people with chronic pain, it's very important that you tense your muscles *gently*—don't strain or cause yourself pain. Tense and release the muscle groups in this order.

1. Toes and feet (curl toes)
2. Calf muscles (push heels down)
3. Thighs
4. Buttocks (clench)
5. Stomach (contract core muscles)
6. Hands and fingers (make fists)
7. Arms
8. Shoulders (shrug)
9. Jaw (clench)
10. Face (scowl)

You can find a recording of this exercise at AftonHassett.com (Resources).

Make It Part of Your Thriving Plan

Follow the prompts above daily or a few times a week. To make PMR or another relaxation technique a habit, set a reminder to practice it at the same time each day. Many people find PMR a great way to ensure a good night's sleep.

DAY 3

MINDFUL BREATHING

DOMAINS: RELAXATION, BETTER SLEEP, ADAPTIVE THOUGHTS

When mindful, you are fully aware of where you are, with whom you're talking, and what you're doing and feeling in the moment, fully present. It feels very different from racing back to a regretful moment in the past or worrying about a possible problem in the future. When mindful, you aren't overreacting to or feeling overwhelmed by what's happening inside you (thoughts and emotions) or around you. You can tune out, dismiss, or ignore the noise. You also recognize that your thoughts and feelings aren't you. They just are and, as such, they can float by like fluffy clouds on a summer day. They don't require your attention.

Given our often busy and noisy minds, mindful awareness sounds challenging. Yet with a little practice, you will get better at staying in the moment and reaping the benefits of feeling relaxed and focused. This technique uses breathing a little differently than on Day 1. We're not trying to breathe slowly, instead we focus on how we're breathing naturally.

Try It Today

These instructions come from *Full Catastrophe Living* by Jon Kabat-Zinn, founder of mindfulness-based stress reduction (MBSR).

- Sit comfortably in a quiet place without disturbances. Close your eyes if you like.
- Pay attention to your stomach. As you breathe, note how your stomach rises and falls.
- Focus on your breathing. Allow yourself to experience each breath, in and out, for its full duration. Ride the waves of breathing as your stomach rises and falls.
- When your mind wanders, note what pulled your attention from your breath, then gently return to the rising and falling of your stomach. Be compassionate with yourself if your attention wanders even a thousand times. That's normal. Simply bring yourself back to your breath. If pain intrudes, notice it without judgment, anger, or fear. It just is. Allow your thoughts about your pain to fade away like mist and return your focus to your breathing.
- Try this exercise for ten minutes. The more your attention wanders the better, because that gives you an excellent starting point for improvement!
- There is a recording for practicing Mindful Breathing at Afton Hassett.com (Resources).

Make It Part of Your Thriving Plan

You can do Mindful Breathing daily or several times a week. You can also practice other mindfulness techniques, such as a Body Scan. To give that method a try, go to PainGuide.com (click on Pain Care, then Self Care, Relaxation, and then, Body Scan).

DAY 4

GUIDED IMAGERY

DOMAINS: RELAXATION, BETTER SLEEP, POSITIVE EMOTIONS

Guided imagery invites you to picture a variety of pleasant scenarios, such as walking down a forest path, watching waves crash on a sandy beach, or snuggling up in your favorite chair with a warm drink. Whatever the scene, the goal is to achieve calm and relaxation.

If asked to describe how you imagine something, visualization likely would come up first. But that's only part of the process. Like your real-world experience, your imagination can have five senses, too. With guided imagery, you can imagine seeing, hearing, smelling, touching, and tasting different details to create a richer, more immersive experience. In addition to pleasant places, guided imagery can provide specific suggestions to help you feel more comfortable or calm. Studies have shown that it helps people with acute or chronic pain, sleep problems, anxiety and depression, healthy eating, and to even boost the immune system.

Try It Today

Guided imagery typically involves listening to recordings. You can find some on AftonHassett.com (Resources) and others at PainGuide.com (Pain Care, Self-Care, Relaxation, Guided Imagery). Several apps have endless options. The content on Insight Timer is excellent, and both the app and access to the recordings are free! Here are some tips:

- In a quiet place where you won't be disturbed, sit comfortably or lie down. Make sure the room feels neither too hot nor too cold and that you can dim the lights. Now listen to your recording. (Never practice this technique while driving!)
- It's normal and expected for your mind to wander. When it does, gently return to the moment and the recording. Maintaining focus and being mindful take practice.
- If you have a hard time engaging all your senses, that's OK, too. Try focusing on just one or two senses; vision and hearing tend to be easiest to imagine. Everyone's different, so note how you imagine details.

Make It Part of Your Thriving Plan

Start with ten or fifteen minutes a day but consider even shorter recordings for first thing in the morning or during work breaks, and longer recordings right before bedtime. Eventually work up to twenty to thirty minutes per day or longer a few times a week. Experiment for a while to see what works best for you.

DAY 5

SAVORING

DOMAINS: POSITIVE EMOTIONS, RELAXATION,

ADAPTIVE THOUGHTS

Savoring just means actively enjoying life's beautiful moments, large and small. Our brains dwell on threats and negative events easily because that process has inherent survival value. In contrast, positive events require more effort to encode in our memories. These stored happy experiences can help you navigate rough times by acting as a buffer. Savoring highlights positive events in the moment, which makes them richer and stickier, so your brain files them away properly.

One of the best ways to savor something as it happens is to engage all your senses. For example, if the event you want to savor is a special moment with someone you love, first recognize that this moment is indeed special. Note in detail how you feel. Is there love, joy, connection, calm, inspiration, or maybe all the above? What do you see? What is the other person wearing? Are flowers growing nearby or birds flying in the sky? What do you hear? Take in the tone of the other person's voice, a radio playing nearby, or the sound of rushing water. What do you smell? Is someone cooking something nearby? What else do you feel in the environment? A cool breeze or warm sunshine? What do you taste? Are you drinking coffee or eating something delicious? These details create a rich mental picture, a complete memory that you can savor in the moment and recall and enjoy again in the future.

Try It Today

It's easy to start with food. During a meal today, identify a dish or ingredient that you really enjoy and savor it for two minutes. Try the following with a favorite dessert.

- Pause to experience and enjoy what you're eating with all five of your senses.
- How does it look? Try to find a detail you might never have noticed before.
- What do you hear? Are you eating something fizzy or crunchy? Is music playing softly in the background?
- How does it smell? Do particular scents contribute to it, such as spices like cinnamon or undertones of other foods like lemon, salt, sugar, or butter?
- Does it feel hot or cold? What texture does it have? Is it smooth or crispy?
- How does it taste? As you chew, breathe in through your nose. Can you detect even more subtle flavors?
- Add an emotion. Are you feeling content, excited, nostalgic, or maybe safe?

Make It Part of Your Thriving Plan

You can savor absolutely anything that brings you joy. Try to savor one pleasant experience every day. Start, if you like, with mindful eating. For your next meal and perhaps more after that, follow the prompts above. Try taking smaller bites and pausing between bites. Appreciate your food from beginning to end. Breathe. Pause. Mindful eating not only improves your mood but can lead to eating a lot less food.

DAY 6

HEALTHY SLEEP HABITS

DOMAINS: BETTER SLEEP, RELAXATION

In Chapter 8, we discussed the importance of sleep and the role it can play in your pain and other symptoms. Hopefully since reading that chapter, you've taken steps to improve your sleep habits. Let's revisit the checklist and see where you are. Check all that apply.

- ☐ I make sleep a priority.
- ☐ Every morning, I wake around the same time, even on weekends.
- ☐ I go to bed close to the same time each night, even on weekends.
- ☐ During the day, I get lots of sunlight, especially in the morning.
- ☐ I consume no caffeine (including chocolate) within ten hours of bedtime.
- ☐ I limit my alcohol intake and drink none within a couple hours of bedtime.
- ☐ I follow a set nightly routine (put on pajamas, stretch, brush teeth, read for thirty minutes).
- ☐ Half an hour before bedtime, I dim the lights.
- ☐ I avoid all electronics for at least thirty to sixty minutes before I go to bed.

☐ I wind down with relaxing activities thirty minutes before bed.

☐ I go to bed only when feeling sleepy.

☐ My bedroom is quiet, cool, and pleasant.

☐ When I turn off the lights, my bedroom is dark, including no glow from an alarm clock.

☐ My pillows and bed feel comfortable.

☐ My bed is only for sleep and sex (no TV, work, bill paying).

☐ Before bed, I use relaxation techniques such as taking slow breaths, PMR, or visualizing a beautiful scene.

☐ I practice gratitude before I close my eyes.

☐ If I don't fall asleep right away, I don't lie in bed worrying or watching the clock. Instead I go do something pleasant but not stimulating until I feel sleepy.

☐ My healthcare provider has reviewed the timing of my medications, and I take them in ways that will enhance sleep.

☐ If I nap, I never do so for more than twenty minutes.

Try It Today

Well, how'd you do? Did you check almost all the healthy sleep habits? If you didn't, pick one or more to start tonight. The first three are the most important.

- Enact the change and see how it works and whether you like it.
- Bonus: Try a modified version of Paced Breathing from Day 1. For falling asleep, count slow breaths backward from thirty to zero to help you relax and drift off.

Make It Part of Your Thriving Plan

Keep following the healthy sleep practices above. Try ranking them, starting with the simple or easy ones to change, and keep at it for two weeks. To aid your practice, check out Insight Timer, a free app loaded with guided imagery recordings, breathing practices, calming meditations, and recordings created specifically to help you sleep better.

DAY 7

TIME-BASED PACING

DOMAIN: PHYSICAL ACTIVITY

We learned a bit about time-based pacing in Chapter 9. This excellent strategy can help you engage in many activities more successfully because you take a break *before* triggering a pain flare-up. People with chronic pain often do an activity until it hurts too much, which can make pain feel worse for days afterwards! For time-based pacing, you'll develop a manageable schedule that alternates activity with rest. You want to identify a safe amount of time that you can do something, then stop *before* the pain flares. You determine the length of time, whether half an hour for something easy or minutes for something a little more challenging. After you take a break, you return to the activity again for another safe amount of time, then rest again. This strategy might take a little longer, but it's a better way of accomplishing tasks without paying dearly in the hours or days that follow.

Here's an example. Let's say you want to do some gardening. Based on prior experience, you know you can garden pain-free for ten or fifteen minutes. So your pacing cycle begins with ten minutes of gardening. Maybe you don't know how long to make your break, so try half the time that you spend active, in this case: five minutes. After resting, try a gentle stretch, garden again for ten more minutes, then take another five-minute break. Repeat this pattern until you finish the activity or task or feel that you need a longer break. That's it!

Try It Today

Activity pacing can apply to almost any task or activity, but it does require some initial guesswork (trial and error).

- Identify the activity or task you want to do. Choose something that you can do right now or later today.
- Think back to the last time you did this activity. How long could you do it without causing a flare? It's OK to have a little dull, achy pain, the type that improves with movement. You don't want to trigger anything sharp or severe, though.
- Select a rest time and determine how you will spend it, for example: sitting, standing, or stretching.
- Set a timer (oven, smartwatch, smartphone, voice-enabled home hub, whatever works best), perform the task, and follow the time limits you've set. If the activity becomes painful, stop immediately and rest even if you didn't reach the time limit.

To aid your practice, PainGuide.com has an excellent module that can help you better understand and practice this technique (click on Pain Care, then Self Care, and Pacing).

Make It Part of Your Thriving Plan

You can pace just about any activity (task, chore, hobby, or sport). Try one or two new activities per week and, if you like, create a log of them so you can track and evaluate your progress.

PLEASANT ACTIVITY SCHEDULING

DOMAINS: POSITIVE EMOTIONS, PHYSICAL ACTIVITY,
MEANING AND PURPOSE, SOCIAL CONNECTIONS

When was the last time you did something *fun*? Because chronic pain greatly limits time and energy, many people spend those precious, limited resources on tasks that *must* be done. So bills, caregiving, chores, errands, and work take priority. Suddenly the day's over, or you've run out of energy, and anything you *like* to do has to wait for another day. Living like that isn't sustainable because a life without joy isn't much of a life. It can create a cycle where not doing what you like or value can lead to feeling *meh* or even depressed. The more you languish, the worse you feel, and, at some point, you lose even the desire to do anything fun or meaningful. What's the solution? Make pleasant activities a priority at least a couple of times a week. This well-studied, disarmingly simple strategy gives you a powerful behavioral tool for countering chronic pain and depression. So, let's have some fun!

Try It Today

- Make a list of ten pleasant activities or tasks that you like to do. They don't need to be big, take extensive planning, or cost a lot of money.

Think about life's simple pleasures, including playing with your kids or pets, working on your hobby, having lunch with a good friend, reading a book, or spending time in nature. Also consider something a little more ambitious such as going to the movies, visiting a museum, attending a concert, or trying a new restaurant. Maybe add one or two big-ticket items, such as a trip somewhere special, that you can plan to do down the road.

- Pick something from your list that you *love* and can do today.
- Select a time to do it and commit to doing it. If it turns out you absolutely can't do it today, pick a time later this week and put it on your calendar.
- When the time comes, don't postpone it. Treat this pleasant activity with the same seriousness as a doctor's appointment!
- While doing the activity, savor it (Day 5). Delight in taking care of yourself. If it becomes a memorable moment, take a photo, buy or pick up a memento, or find another way to commemorate the happy experience.

Make It Part of Your Thriving Plan

Schedule two or three activities a week, every week. You don't need to invest a lot of time in them. Often just thirty minutes will suffice. At the end of the days that include one of the pleasant activities, focus on what it was like and how good it made you feel. No guilt allowed—this is part of your long-term pain management program.

DAY 9

WALKING PROGRAM

DOMAINS: PHYSICAL ACTIVITY, SOCIAL
CONNECTIONS, BETTER SLEEP

This activity could be one of the best things you can do to improve your pain, your mood, and your life. Your brain needs physical exercise as does the rest of your body. According to the National Institutes of Health, walking improves heart health, regulates blood pressure, benefits circulation, strengthens muscles, increases lung capacity, reduces stress, supports weight loss, and helps you feel happier! As a form of exercise, walking doesn't require a gym membership or special equipment, and you can do it throughout the day. If you have no problems with walking in general, you probably can start without asking a doctor first, but it never hurts to ask. Definitely check with your healthcare provider if you feel dizzy, short of breath, or faint when walking. Also, talk to your physician beforehand if you have a heart condition, high blood pressure, diabetes, or have been inactive for a long time.

To stay healthy, adults should aim for at least 150 minutes of moderate-intensity aerobic activity each week, or about twenty minutes per day. Brisk walking qualifies as moderate intensity because it raises your heart rate.

You're walking quickly, but you still should be able to breathe and carry on a conversation. Are you game?

Try It Today

Plan a brisk walk for ten minutes today. You can start with less time if you need or more time if you want. If you would like to use steps as your guide, about 1,000 steps will work—for the walk, not for the whole day.

- Wear comfortable shoes with good support and appropriate clothing.
- If walking outdoors, grab your phone, keys, and identification. It's never a bad idea to let someone know where you're going.
- Choose an easy, flat, scenic route if possible.
- Start slowly and let your body warm up.
- Keep your chin up, maintain good posture, and swing your arms freely.
- After a few minutes, try a gentle stretch if you like.
- Increase your pace for the rest of your session.
- At the end, slow your pace, allow your breathing to return to normal, and try another gentle stretch.
- Pat yourself on the back and take note of your time and/or steps.

Make It Part of Your Thriving Plan

After today, I would love for you to continue this activity throughout the thirty-day exploration period and beyond. Almost everyone can benefit from a walking program, and it could be a foundational element of your long-term plan. Increase your sessions by one minute or 100 steps per day. Walking with a friend or group adds a great social component to the practice. Companionship, encouragement, and accountability can help on days when you feel less motivated. If you have a dog, the two of you can head out together. See who can spot more squirrels along the way!

TAKE A NATURE BREAK

DOMAINS: RELAXATION, PHYSICAL ACTIVITY, POSITIVE EMOTIONS, MEANING AND PURPOSE

Until relatively recently, we humans spent most of our time outdoors: roaming forests, meadows, and jungles, surrounded by greenery, sun, wind, flowing water, and birdsong. (Bet you didn't know that birdsong can have positive health effects![104]) Now we constrict ourselves with concrete, bricks, steel, glass, pavement, and noise. No wonder we feel so stressed. We all need a little nature exposure at least a few times a week. Spending time in nature has health benefits for people with chronic pain, migraines, depression, anxiety, obesity, diabetes, cardiovascular disease, various infectious diseases, cancer, respiratory disease, healing after surgery, and attention-deficit/hyperactivity disorder (ADHD).

Try It Today

You don't need to spend a week camping in the forest to reap nature's health benefits. Just get outside, find some trees, plants, or grass, and engage your senses. Here's how.

- Plan how you will access nature. If you live in the suburbs or a more rural area, no sweat. Go to a nearby forest, meadow, mountain, or beach. If you live in a city, visit green spaces such as parks, riverbanks, or even an open academic campus with greenery (and outdoor seating). If you have outdoor space in the city, such as a balcony or even just one planter, fill it with local plants and flowers.
- Studies indicate that two hours spent enjoying nature seems to be the right "dose." If that's not possible, aim for twenty or thirty minutes.
- If the weather looks lousy, gaze out the window at the nearest green spaces or put on a nature documentary.

Make It Part of Your Thriving Plan

Just go outside! Immerse yourself in some aspect of nature every day. Take in all the shapes and colors, listen to the birds or other animals, smell the flowers or plants, feel the sun or wind on your face, and taste a piece of fresh fruit that you brought with you. The key is to mindfully take it all in—set your phone aside and be in the moment.

SHOW YOURSELF COMPASSION

DOMAINS: ADAPTIVE THOUGHTS, POSITIVE EMOTIONS

For the next few days, we're going to spend some time thinking about thinking, with the goal of you choosing an adaptive thought strategy for your Thriving Plan. Whatever approach you pick, all helpful or more adaptive thoughts work in a similar way. Adaptive thoughts calm you emotionally and physically, dialing down the brain's perceived threat level and its explosion of emotional activity (remember amygdala hijack?). With this moment of peace, you can engage the reasoning parts of your brain before you react.

Coping thoughts also spark positive emotions. They make you think more creatively, make decisions more effectively, and help you feel more optimistic. Whatever approach(es) you choose, the best road to success starts with a healthy dose of self-compassion, defined by Kristin Neff at the University of Texas at Austin as "how we relate to ourselves in instances of perceived failure, inadequacy, or personal suffering." The idea is as simple as giving yourself the same kindness and care that you'd give to a good friend.

Try It Today

- Think about a time you failed, made a big mistake, had a major setback, or experienced a bad situation that you think you made worse.
- What happened? Use pen and paper or your computer to write about the event in as much detail as you can recall.
- Next, draw or type a line and, below that, list all the thoughts you have about the incident and your role in it.
- After that, draw or type another line and describe how your thoughts about this event make you feel.
- Now, pretend your best friend just told you the same story as though it happened to him or her.
- What would you say in response? Draw or type another line and write that down. Are you saying something different to your friend than yourself? If so, how does it differ?
- Take a deep breath and show yourself a moment of compassion. Tell yourself exactly what you would have told your friend—and *mean it*.
- What have you learned, and how can you show yourself more compassion in the future?

Make It Part of Your Thriving Plan

Self-compassion takes practice, and the people most in need of it usually don't believe they deserve it. When your inner critic starts beating you down, step aside from that ugly word storm and channel what you'd tell your friend instead.

THOUGHT APPROACH 1: REFRAME NEGATIVE THOUGHTS

DOMAIN: ADAPTIVE THOUGHTS

Cognitive behavioral therapy (CBT) helps people identify and change unhelpful thoughts. We all have them. Some of them grew from childhood experiences, our culture, the media, and elsewhere. Whatever the source, they generally just pop into your head without warning, undermining your ability to be successful and happy. Newsflash! You don't need to accept them without question. Please, question them. The skill of *reframing* helps change the most unhelpful, pessimistic, irrational, and catastrophic thoughts into those that can help us act more confidently and feel less gloomy or helpless. Your thoughts have incredible power. Replacing overly negative ones can give you a fresh, more realistic perspective on life.

Try It Today

- Identify an overly negative thought. Most of them involve an absolute, such as: *all, always, everyone, everything, forever, never, no one, nothing,* and *only.* Examples include: *There's* nothing *I can* ever *do to ease my pain;* everyone *thinks I'm a failure;* and *I* always *make a fool of myself.* These catastrophic thoughts evoke negative emotions, and negative behaviors soon follow (avoidance, inactivity, procrastination, self-sabotage).

- Challenge the negative thought. What hard evidence or proof do you have that it's 100 percent true? Gather evidence that supports the negative thought and evidence that refutes it as a bunch of hooey. Let's take *There's nothing I can ever do to ease my pain*. The evidence in favor might include that, on some days, nothing seems to help. The evidence against it recognizes that, on most days, you usually can do a few things to ease the pain. There, you've challenged the negative thought!

- Develop a new, better thought by focusing on the evidence that you used to disprove the negative thought. For the example case, the better, replacement thought might be: *Most days I can make my pain a little better*. Realistic thoughts tend to run longer and have more nuance, but so what. They not only are more accurate, but they also are much less distressing, which encourages you to engage in more healthy behaviors.

Make It Part of Your Thriving Plan

If you want to develop this skill as part of your long-term pain management plan, star this page, then check out PainGuide.com (click on Pain Care, Self-Care, Reframing) for more information and helpful tools you can use to practice reframing overly negative thoughts. It takes some practice but this skill can change your life in remarkable ways!

THOUGHT APPROACH 2: UNHELPFUL THOUGHTS COME AND GO

DOMAIN: ADAPTIVE THOUGHTS

Why do we suffer? Maybe it's because we're too smart for our own good. According to Steven Hayes, creator of acceptance and commitment therapy (ACT), our ability to plan, predict, evaluate, connect, solve, and communicate elevates our status in the pecking order among species, but that sophisticated use of language and complex thought also leaves us vulnerable to suffering and misery. We expect to be able to control our thoughts and feelings just like we can control what we have for breakfast.

As a core principle, ACT helps disentangle us from negative thoughts. It takes a little practice, but we can learn to recognize that our thoughts are not us. They are separate from us. Let's take the thought, *I'll never do anything meaningful because of my pain.* If you had this thought and believed it, you might never try to do anything meaningful. But could you simply notice this thought and step away from it like watching a dandelion seed float on the breeze? If we try to escape our thoughts by dulling them with substances or denying their existence, we set ourselves up for failure. Instead, try allowing your thoughts to simply exist. Thoughts are, after all, just a bunch of concepts, ideas, or images—inanimate, abstract objects, really—that have no power over you *unless you give them power.* We sometimes forget that we don't need to believe or act on everything that pops into our heads. If we did, chaos would ensue! Accept that thoughts happen, emotions happen, and lousy events happen.

Try It Today

- Sit peacefully and invite your inner critic to share an opinion or two about you. When something unpleasant pops into your head, write it down. Let's consider this thought.
- Is this a single clear thought, or is it a jumble of several thoughts? If a jumble, tighten it into one clear sentence, like the example above: *I'll never do anything meaningful because of my pain.* That's a good one, full of negativity and absolutes.
- Sit with your negative thought for a bit. Maybe say it aloud.
- Now consider your thought scientifically. Add the phrase, "I'm having this thought that—" in front of it. So, for our example: *I'm having this thought that I'll never do anything meaningful because of my pain.*
- Note the mental shift that took place when you did that. In an instant, you shifted from hosting a damning indictment of yourself to examining a clump of words passing through your mind.
- Breathe in and then exhale while imagining the thought exiting your mind and floating away like a leaf on the breeze.

Make It Part of Your Thriving Plan

Conjure, appraise, and release at least one negative thought per day. To expand your practice of ACT for chronic pain, check out the great book by Dahl and Lundgren listed in the Resources section of this book (page 255).

THOUGHT APPROACH 3: COPING COACH

DOMAIN: ADAPTIVE THOUGHTS

You can act as your own wellness coach. When armed with solid coping thoughts, you can navigate stressful situations far more effectively than when you let negative thoughts dictate your options and self-image. You likely already know lots of great coping thoughts because you say them to other people faced with adversity. More optimistic, and often more realistic, coping thoughts make you more likely to act instead of bogging you down in avoidance, fear, and procrastination. Here are some examples. Read each line slowly, pause, and note how you feel.

> Unhelpful: *I can't stand it any longer!*
> Coping: *It's hard, but I can ride it out one moment at a time.*
> Unhelpful: *I'm so pathetic. I'll never be able to do this.*
> Coping: *I'm more capable and stronger than I think.*

Coping thoughts work in many ways. First, they calm you down. They dial down that amygdala hijack surge of negative emotions and even spark positive ones. At the same time, muscle tension decreases, and you're

DAY 15

THOUGHT APPROACH 4:
SOMATIC TRACKING

DOMAINS: ADAPTIVE THOUGHTS, POSITIVE EMOTIONS

Pain reprocessing therapy (PRT) acknowledges that the brain constantly processes countless bits of incoming information and must screen out almost all of it, including breathing, itches, heartbeat, and pulse. The brain can attend only to a few bits of information at a time. You pay attention to what draws your attention, and potential threats draw attention most effectively. When the brain constantly is scanning for threats, it will find them even if the physical sensation turns out to be completely harmless. Once that harmless sensation is misinterpreted as threat, you likely will experience pain.[105] Your brain has become an overprotective nanny screaming at you to stop, withdraw, and avoid all activities, situations, and people for fear of injury. Great. So what can you do? PRT offers an effective skill called somatic tracking, which aims to teach you how to consider painful sensations through the lens of safety. Let's give it a try.

more likely to make healthy choices, all of which serves to make your pain better.

Try It Today

- Identify a few key thoughts that have proven helpful in the past, thoughts that have calmed you down. Also think back to advice you've given other people to help them handle adversity.
- List thoughts specific to you and your experiences. For example, if you avoid certain activities for fear you might (re)injure yourself, a coping thought would be, *My doctor encourages me to exercise and has told me I'm ready.*
- Choose positive coping thoughts that ring true, for example: *People in my life love and support me* rings more truthful and realistic than *Everyone loves me and supports me.*
- Come up with a few short, appealing coping mantras for when you feel stressed or upset: *I am loved. This too shall pass. Breathe and achieve. Fierce and feisty. I got this*—whatever resonates with you.
- Write these coping mantras on sticky notes and place them where you can see them, add them to your calendar as a recurring event, or engrave your mantra on a small medallion and wear it around your neck. Make them easy to remember and easy to spot when you need them.

Make It Part of Your Thriving Plan

Recite the adaptive thoughts when you wake up, before you go to bed, and any time you need a little extra boost of confidence. Aim to catch negative thoughts as they happen and coach yourself with supportive advice.

Try It Today

As with every skill in this book, seek confirmation from your healthcare provider that tissue injury *hasn't* caused your pain and that movement is safe. If this is the case, your pain is a prime target for somatic tracking.

- Identify one physical position or activity that tends to elicit pain, perhaps sitting, standing, bending, twisting, or climbing stairs.
- Don your scientist hat and mindfully explore your pain sensation with openness, interest, and curiosity. Start with the idea that you don't need to stop or change the pain; just consider it. Does it feel sharp or dull? Does it exist in one location or many? How intense does it feel, and does that change as you consider it? If it were a color, what color would it be?
- Now, put on your "safety goggles" and consider that painful sensation from the perspective that it represents *no potential harm*. Your doctor has assured you of this already. Tissue or bone damage isn't causing your pain—it's just a signal like thousands of other benign signals your brain is attending to or ignoring. You can pay attention to that signal or focus on an itch, your heartbeat, the sun on your face, or some music.
- The goal is to focus your attention on more positive thoughts and sensations. Invite positive images and emotions to flow. Picture yourself on the happiest day of your life, plan a fun outing for later in the day or week, or focus on a pleasant sensation in your body, such as a soft fabric on your skin.

Make It Part of Your Thriving Plan

You can practice this skill with different painful sensations throughout the day, every day. Eventually your brain will stop perceiving the painful sensations as potential threats, then they can recede into the background, ignored like all the other benign signals (eye blinking, pulse, left shoe tied a bit too tight) your brain chooses to ignore. If you'd like to explore this approach further, check out the books by Alan Gordon and Howard Schubiner in the Resources section of this book (page 255).

SELF-SOOTHE

DOMAINS: RELAXATION, ADAPTIVE THOUGHTS

When feeling intensely emotional, we rarely act in productive ways. We *react* and sometimes say and do things we regret. The power to use higher-order thinking, including logic and restraint, escapes us when we're freaking out (amygdala hijack). When in a frenzied state, we first need to calm down so our thinking brain can wrest control back from our emotional brain. A form of CBT, dialectical behavior therapy (DBT) has provided some excellent techniques for calming and restoring sanity.[106] One approach for dampening intense emotions calls for relying on your senses. Primitive and powerful, our senses existed before language. You already might know which senses tend to make you feel better. For example, when stressed, you might soothe yourself with comfort food (taste), a warm shower (touch), aromatherapy (smell), music (hearing), or a sunset (sight). Whichever sounds most familiar will give you a hint as to what sense(s) to engage when life goes sideways.

Try It Today

Consider each of the senses and activities that follow. Many people with chronic pain have sensory sensitivity, so what might smell delightful to one person seems like an assault on the nose to another. This principle holds true for all the senses, so pursue what sounds best to you.

- Vision, perhaps your most complex and distracting sense, can be calming. Watch a sunrise, clouds floating by, a sunset, or stars in the sky. Select a flower, plant, or tree and contemplate every aspect of it. Find photos of the most beautiful places on earth. In an online museum, identify your favorite pieces of art.
- Many sounds enhance relaxation. Listen to a favorite piece of music; a recording of rain, waves crashing on a beach, a babbling brook; or a podcast or audiobook discussing a joyful or peaceful topic. Go outside and listen for birdsong and other sounds of nature.
- A powerful sense, smell can transport you to moments when you felt calm and safe. To delight your nose, put on a favorite lotion or cologne; light a scented candle or burn some incense; slice open a lemon, lime, or orange and rub its oils on your skin; or open a package of coffee or tea and breathe in deeply.
- Given that you live with chronic pain, your sense of touch matters. Wrap yourself in a fluffy blanket or a pile of warm clothes fresh from the dryer. Take a soothing bath and consider adding a foaming bath bomb. Pet a cat, dog, hamster, horse, or rabbit. For stressful situations, touch a stuffed animal or piece of soft, velvety fabric that instantly puts you at ease.
- To engage taste, which also closely ties to memory, slowly eat a handful of raisins; drink a cup of tea, hot chocolate, or decaf coffee; let a small piece of chocolate melt on your tongue; or suck on a tart candy or chew some minty gum.

Make It Part of Your Thriving Plan

After you've tried all the above activities over time, identify which ones work best for you. Then prepare an emergency checklist or kit to help calm yourself when you most need it.

DAY 17

RELEASE PAINFUL EMOTIONS

DOMAINS: ADAPTIVE THOUGHTS, RELAXATION

A powerful strategy, letting go of negative emotions can help you gain better control over them and yourself. The foundation of this skill rests on what we learned for Day 13, allowing negative thoughts to come and go without judgment or dread. To let go of negative emotions, first begin by accepting that you have them. We all do, but we often find ourselves ashamed of our shame, angry at our anger, or depressed that we're sad. When you judge your emotions harshly and tell yourself you just should be happy, it makes you more likely to wallow in them, bury them, or dismiss their potential value instead of understanding them and letting them pass like clouds fading across the sky. Today we're going to try another skill that also comes from DBT, which involves the central idea that acceptance *isn't* approval. Everyone can have ugly emotions, but just because you understand that you're having them doesn't mean they get to have you. When you can name and accept that you're having a negative emotion, it loses power over you. You don't need to judge yourself harshly for having it. Fighting yourself makes you weaker and the emotion stronger—not at all what we want!

Try It Today

- Whatever the emotion may be and whenever it hits, just consider it for a moment. Does it contain any objectively important information? If so, contemplate that information dispassionately. Then proceed with the rest of the steps.
- *Identify the emotion.* Acknowledge that you're experiencing it and give it a name: anger, fear, sadness, jealousy, shame, disappointment, hatred, and so on.
- *Connect the emotion.* Think about it from a distance like a scientist. *How interesting that I'm feeling this emotion.* Where did it come from? Can you connect it to what you were just thinking? Can you connect it to how your pain feels right now?
- *Feel the emotion.* Let it build, crest, then fizzle like an ocean wave breaking on the shore. Breathe. Don't push the emotion away, which only will make it sneakier. Don't judge it either, which only will make it more powerful.
- *Accept and Reset.* You exist separately from this emotion. It simply is. Don't judge it or yourself. Remember, *acceptance isn't approval*, and you don't need to act on the emotion. Just acknowledge it and let it go. Pick an image such as a drifting cloud, a big red balloon floating away, crumpling a piece of paper and throwing it in the recycling bin, or fat, soapy bubbles popping. That's the negative emotion, which you've diminished.

Make It Part of Your Thriving Plan

First remember the words: Identify, Connect, Feel, Accept, Reset (ICFAR). Then create a reminder to help walk you through this exercise, ending with the visual metaphor—cloud, balloon, paper, bubble—that resonates with you most. Here, too, keeping a journal can help you track your emotions and how they impact your pain.

EMBRACE POSITIVE EMOTIONS

DOMAINS: POSITIVE EMOTIONS, MEANING
AND PURPOSE, ADAPTIVE THOUGHTS

The brains of people with chronic pain can have difficulty processing positive occurrences and emotions. It's kind of like losing your sense of taste, a common problem for people with COVID. If you can't appreciate food, you lose the desire to eat it or even seek it. The same principle holds true for positive emotions in many people with chronic pain. The good news is that, like losing your sense of taste due to illness, it almost always comes back. Learning to detect and appreciate positive emotions requires a little brain retraining. Even if just for today, keep a positive piggy bank. This activity can remind you to focus on the good moments in your day and seek more positive people, events, and experiences. Not all positive events should hit the peak of a luxury vacation or a new car. What tends to make us happiest are small occurrences such as a pleasant conversation with a friend, a melty chocolate chip cookie, or a walk in nature.

Try It Today

The instructions below show you how to keep a positive piggy bank for today.

- Select a jar, small box, or a piggy bank that makes you smile and put it somewhere that you'll see it, such as on the kitchen counter or by your bed.
- Place small slips of paper (three-by-three-inch sticky notes work well) and a pen by your container.
- Every evening, think about the positive people, events, or experiences from that day, someone or something that brought you a moment of peace, a feeling of gratitude, or made you laugh or smile.
- Pick one and spend a moment savoring it. Think about what made it so special to you.
- Write down the happy occurrence using enough detail to help you recall it later.
- Fold your positive memory and drop it in the container.

Make It Part of Your Thriving Plan

Now that you have set up a Positive Piggy Bank, why not keep it going? Make one positive memory deposit in the same way every evening. You choose how long you want to do this: one week, two weeks, one month, or longer. Shake the container and make withdrawals any time you need them. Try waiting a couple of weeks between withdrawals and reading the happy memories all at once, recalling in detail what made them so special to you.

MUSIC IS EMOTIONAL MEDICINE

DOMAINS: POSITIVE EMOTIONS, MEANING
AND PURPOSE, RELAXATION

Music is such a meaningful part of our lives. It profoundly can affect how we feel, what we remember, and even what we do. Think about it: Have you ever felt a little low and then you hear a great song, and you can't stop your feet from tapping, your hips from swaying, or your lips from smiling? Other songs can trigger powerful waves of nostalgia or memories good or bad. Even people who have hearing impairments perceive rhythmic vibration in the same parts of the brain as those used for processing sound in hearing individuals. Feeling music provides a similar experience, and the development of new wearable technology can translate music into full-body vibration. So music is primal, powerful, and universal. It can improve your mood and decrease your pain, and it's right at your fingertips! You can enjoy music in so many ways that it might feel difficult to choose the best way to bring more of it into your life. If you love music, make it part of your long-term Thriving Plan to help you experience less pain, feel happier, function better, and connect with others.

Try It Today

- For today, select and listen to just two or three songs or pieces of music that make you feel invincible, proud, optimistic, or strong; any genre—classical, jazz, rock, pop, alternative, country, electronic, hip hop, R&B, whatever you love. When you hear these songs, they should make you feel good. Crank up the volume and get into it!

Make It Part of Your Thriving Plan

If music makes you feel better, let's explore some different ways to engage in music therapeutically. Try one or more of these ideas for your Thriving Plan.

- Assemble a soundtrack. Identify your favorite songs from the best times in your life. Consider summer songs, dance music, movie soundtracks, show tunes, sports chants, Motown, or whatever brings you joy.
- Create a playlist. There are so many (changing) ways to access music and build your own playlists that I could never do justice to listing them all. Go old-school, bust out your old records, tapes, or CDs, and make a mix or assemble one to stream on a mobile device.
- Go live! Attend as many in-person performances or concerts as you can. Don't forget to consider free events, too, such as jazz in the park, coffeehouse showcases, school choirs, gospel or other religious music at church, recitals at your local college, and even public libraries, which are curating more live music.
- Make your own kind of music. If you love to sing, sing. If you love to play an instrument, go get it and noodle away. Enjoy writing songs? Do more of that. Just want to tap on some drums or other percussion instruments to feel the rhythm and vibration in your body? Go for it!

DAY 20

CREATE A RELATIONSHIP TREE

DOMAINS: SOCIAL CONNECTIONS, MEANING AND PURPOSE

As we learned in the chapter on social relationships, feeling connected and a sense of belonging can help you feel happier, healthier, and even live longer. Strong positive relationships offer many benefits, but unhealthy ones can make you sadder and sicker. Considering your social circles isn't an easy exercise because you have to be honest with yourself and your own role in whether the relationship feels positive or negative. You need to ask yourself: Does it make sense to make reasonable changes to improve the relationship, such as listening better, communicating feelings more freely, speaking more truthfully, or behaving more considerately? Some relationships are just plain unhealthy, and some people in your life may not have your best interests at heart. For the latter, you don't need to cut them from your life completely—especially when they're related to you—but you may want to focus your precious energy on building relationships that feel more supportive and rewarding.

Try It Today

Building the strongest, healthiest relationship tree possible requires regular thought and action. Today, we simply are going to examine the health of your tree. For this activity, you need some art supplies: paper, pen or pencil, and two or three highlighters of different colors. Crayons or colored pens or pencils work great, too.

- In the bottom third of the paper, draw yourself as the trunk of the tree. It doesn't need to look like you. Just draw a tree trunk.
- For every person in your life, add a leaf either with a leaf shape or a circle containing the person's name. Place the people closest to you or those with whom you spend the most time closest to the trunk. Draw people who play a less active role in your life further up, away from the trunk.
- Be as inclusive as you can. Think about friends, family (close or distant), neighbors, coworkers, schoolmates, fellow spiritual practitioners, hobby buddies, and so on. If you use social media, consider looking through your lists of friends or followers to make sure you're not forgetting anyone important. (If you don't recognize or remember some of them, now might be a good time to do a little digital pruning.)
- Once you feel you have all the meaningful leaves in place, use your highlighters to code the health of different relationships, for example: green for healthy, yellow for neutral, and red for negative.
- When you're done highlighting the health of your social tree, how does it look? Do you see lots of healthy leaves (good relationships) or a bunch of negative ones? Do the positive relationships cluster near the trunk, protecting you from the negative ones further away? Do you see clusters of positive people at home and negative people at work or vice versa?
- Consider each relationship and decide how you want to move forward. Which relationships should you tend and nurture? Which relationships should you try to repair? Which relationships need some additional distance? Which truly unhealthy relationships need to be pruned?

Make It Part of Your Thriving Plan

You can and should tend to your social tree's health for the rest of your life. Who you have in your life and what roles you allow them to play can affect both your happiness and health. Repeat this exercise once or twice a year, perhaps on your birthday and/or New Year's Day.

DAY 21

DAILY CONNECTION

DOMAINS: SOCIAL CONNECTIONS, MEANING AND PURPOSE

After completing the relationship tree exercise, you likely have a much better sense of the relationships that you'd like to nurture. You have the *who*, but what about the *how*? As you know, building healthy and fulfilling relationships takes time and effort. Most people with chronic pain struggle to find the time and energy for valued activities beyond work, errands, and chores. So you'll need a feasible action plan to connect regularly with the people you care about. Today is all about making a habit of daily connection with someone special. Let's discuss three methods: Text to Connect, One More Question, and Heartfelt Compliment.

Try It Today

Choose one of the three ideas below and give it a try.

- *Text to Connect:* Most of us text *a lot*, so this might be the easiest of the bunch. Scroll down your text message list and find someone with whom you have a positive relationship but haven't spoken to in a while. Send the person a warm text saying something to the effect of: "Thinking of you and hope all is well!" Make it personal and meaningful; say whatever makes the most sense in the context of your relationship. That could mean adding a picture of you both, a funny GIF, or a series of emojis, too.

- *One More Question:* Asking people questions shows that you're listening and interested. It's a gift and a skill. Too often we busily think more about how we might respond than absorbing what others are saying. Wow someone with one more question that shows you heard and care. Be fully present with interested eyes and a warm smile.

- *Heartfelt Compliment:* You can demonstrate genuine interest in others by offering compliments about something meaningful to them. It could be a character strength, talent, or achievement that you admire. Also, it might seem a little shallow, but we all like to hear that a new haircut looks nice or that someone thinks our shoes are cool.

Make It Part of Your Thriving Plan

Implement one or all the above activities on a regular basis, say the first of the month, which is easy to remember but not so often that you're trying too much or too hard.

While we're talking about relationships and communicating, let's broach a sensitive topic: how to talk about your illness or chronic pain. Your pain is a part of you. It's loud and bossy and screams for your attention. It makes sense to want to talk to others about it, which is fine and healthy. But focusing only on pain means losing a big piece of who you are beyond your symptoms. Discuss your pain when it comes up in conversation, yes, but remember that you're *so* much more than just your pain!

FORGIVE

DOMAINS: SOCIAL CONNECTIONS, ADAPTIVE THOUGHTS

Country music gives us some of the most candid depictions of the terrible ways that we humans treat one another: lying, cheating, stealing, hurting. Those songs resonate because selfish or senseless acts of awfulness are part of the deal of having other humans in our day-to-day lives. What really counts, though, is how we handle the indiscretions of others. You can hold a big, long, ugly grudge, sure. But grudges typically hurt the holder more than the offender. Holding grudges invites bitterness and suspicion into all your relationships and subjects you to the deleterious health effects of negative emotions and persistent stress. So, we need to try to find a way to forgive. Forgiving doesn't mean excusing, condoning, accepting, or approving the bad behavior of others; it instead releases you from negative thoughts, emotions, and behaviors interfering with your happiness and health. Forgiveness is letting go of unproductive feelings for the sake of your own well-being.

Try It Today

Everitt Worthington, professor emeritus at Virginia Commonwealth University, has conducted pioneering work in this area and offers a path for achieving forgiveness.[107] His REACH model consists of the following basic principles and steps:

- *Recall:* Acknowledge what happened and that you felt hurt. Step back from thoughts of hate or vengeance and commit to the idea of forgiveness.
- *Explore and empathize with the other person:* Put yourself in the other person's shoes. Try to understand what led to the hurtful action—not excusing, just understanding.
- *Altruistic gift:* Remember a time when you received forgiveness for something that you did. You likely felt grateful and motivated to do better. Give your forgiveness as an unselfish, altruistic gift.
- *Commit:* Once you have forgiven someone, make it stick. Perhaps grant it in public or put it in writing.
- *Hold onto forgiveness:* It's easy to slip back into grudges. One way to hold onto your forgiveness would be to write yourself a note to remind you that forgiveness was granted.

For today, choose to forgive just one person, either for a minor transgression—so you can get the hang of it—or, perhaps, choose to work on forgiving a *biggie*. Whatever you decide is fine as long as you choose to grant someone forgiveness today. Follow the steps above.

Make It Part of Your Thriving Plan

If you can, try to forgive one person per month. You could let go of old grudges first and newer ones later or small infractions and then bigger ones. Also remember that you can forgive people no longer in your life for whatever reason, such as distance or death, and you can forgive a person for more than one offense. It's never too late.

We also need to find ways to forgive ourselves. Remember Day 11, when we discussed the importance of self-compassion? That means that you need to cut yourself a little slack, too. A willingness to forgive yourself is paramount to your mental and physical health.

ACTS OF KINDNESS

**DOMAINS: SOCIAL CONNECTIONS, POSITIVE EMOTIONS,
MEANING AND PURPOSE, PHYSICAL ACTIVITY**

As we discussed in Chapter 13, acts of kindness can have a ripple effect, one act inspiring another and so on. Remember, too, that acts of kindness make both parties feel happier. That's a win-win proposition! So what constitutes an act of kindness? Well, some high-effort options include volunteering to build schools or homes for disadvantaged communities, tutoring or teaching a child to read, helping at a food pantry or homeless shelter, bringing meals to homebound people, walking a dog for someone who can't, donating your hair to an organization that makes wigs for people who have hair loss, donating new toys to a children's hospital, and more. But small, everyday kindnesses might have the greatest effect on your health and happiness, the kinds of actions that require little effort or cost nothing, such as paying someone a heartfelt compliment, leaving notes of support to be found, helping a friend with a chore, thanking someone in the military for their service, or giving a loved one a warm hug. Those small but powerful acts will boost your mood as well. Studies have shown that the most effective kindness prescription involves planning and executing five small acts in one day. Let's give that a whirl today.

Try It Today

Plan and do five small kind acts for family members, friends, strangers, society, or the planet.

- Think about what you might want to do. Small acts can include helping a friend in need, holding the door for someone, letting a car merge in front of you in traffic, writing a nice online review for a local independent business, or collecting trash at a park or beach. For more kind acts, visit AftonHassett.com.
- Decide who you want to help. Aim for a combination of people you know and don't know.
- Don't expect anything in return. People unused to kindness, especially if coming from a stranger, might give you quizzical looks or odd reactions.
- Smile as you do your kind act, knowing that you're adding positivity to the world.
- If someone asks what you're doing or why, simply say: "It's just an act of kindness. Please pass it on."
- Extra credit: After you've completed your five kind acts, do one kind thing for yourself. People with chronic pain often put others first and forget to be kind to themselves. To flourish, you must take care of yourself, too. Consider taking a long bath or shower, reading your favorite book or author for a while, or having a special dessert after dinner.

Make It Part of Your Thriving Plan

It doesn't make practical sense to do five acts every single day. Instead, try to do one intentionally kind thing per day for someone else and one for yourself. Alternatively, you could plan a day of kindness per week or per month. Keep the actions small but meaningful, helpful but not financial. In your diary or calendar, consider noting what you did and how it made you feel. Now go spread some kindness!

DAY 24

THE GIFT OF GIVING

DOMAINS: SOCIAL CONNECTIONS, POSITIVE
EMOTIONS, MEANING AND PURPOSE

People love gifts. Remember, in your childhood, that frenzied anticipation of your birthday party or the thrill of festively wrapped holiday packages with your name on them? Even today, most of us are suckers for a small surprise even if it costs little or isn't terribly useful. We like that someone thought of us, took the time to shop or make something, and gave it to us in anticipation that it might make us smile. Even though we like to receive gifts, the wellness benefit often belongs to the giver. That's right, it really is better to give than receive! The gift doesn't need to be tangible, either. It can be an experience. An exceptional dinner, tickets to a game or concert, or visiting someplace exciting can have more positive effects than giving people stuff, even *big* stuff. Experiential gifts can be especially impactful for children who can cherish the memories for a lifetime. So let's give someone something special!

Try It Today

- Think about a person whom you'd like to surprise with a small gift. Imagine what that person might like.

- Now consider some ideas for tangible gifts: a picture frame with a photo of the two of you together; a card containing a meaningful poem or a reference to a shared joke or experience; homemade cookies or a treat from the person's favorite bakery; a chocolate truffle in a fancy box with a bow; a self-care product such as a bath bomb or scented lotion; a book the person expressed interest in reading, containing a warm inscription; a small plant or some wildflowers; or something you made with your hands and heart. Also consider intangible gifts that can bring joy, such as the gift of your time or a donation in someone's name.

- This is perhaps the hardest part of this exercise: give the gift *without expectations*.

Make It Part of Your Thriving Plan

To make this a habit, perhaps pick one day a month on which you'll gift something meaningful to someone you care about. Remember, these small gifts should be thoughtful and don't need to cost much if anything. You might already have what you need (a card in your desk, a photo, a poem), or you easily can pick something up on the way to see them (a book, a treat, a bottle of wine). Do this activity monthly for as long as it brings you joy.

PRACTICE GRATITUDE

DOMAINS: MEANING AND PURPOSE, POSITIVE

EMOTIONS, ADAPTIVE THOUGHTS

Gratitude can include heartfelt appreciation for worldly basics, such as having a home, food to eat, and clean water to drink, as well as thankfulness for life-improving possessions, including transportation, a smartphone, or comfortable shoes. Gratitude for possessions with an emotional connection—a gift from your beloved or an album of irreplaceable family photos—can be particularly powerful. Bigger, less tangible items, such as rewarding friendships; having a good, happy, meaningful day; your loving relationship with your pet; or watching the sunrise or sunset can make you feel warm with gratitude. Feeling a connection to something greater and other spiritual experiences also can yield deep feelings of gratitude. But gratitude usually doesn't just pop into your head out of the blue. Feeling that warm wave flow over you typically requires you to reflect on the people, events, activities, and objects that have meaning for you. You often need to take a moment to express and feel appreciation. But it can be hard to feel grateful when you have chronic pain. When you hurt physically and emotionally, it's much easier to feel angry and resentful. After all, you've lost so much. Still, if you open your heart to the goodness around you, big and small, a moment of gratitude can wash away a bit of the pain. It's very hard to feel grateful and miserable at the same time.

Try It Today

- Watch the TEDx talk "Gratitude" by Louie Schwartzberg.
- Spend a few minutes thinking about the people, things, and simple gifts in your life that you appreciate.
- Write down three big things for which you're grateful and three small things.
- For each thing you wrote down, explain *why* you are grateful for it.
- Read your notes and allow gratitude to wash over you.

Make It Part of Your Thriving Plan

Keeping a gratitude journal can become one of the most rewarding parts of your Thriving Plan. Here's what you can do:

- Your journal can take the form of a new journal bought just for this activity, a small paper notebook, a dedicated gratitude app, a file on your computer, or the notepad on a mobile device.
- Every day, write down two or three things for which you're grateful, big (family, health, home) or small (flowers, ponies, pie).
- Here's the tricky part. What you record each day must be *different*. No repeats! This rule will encourage you to search for different things that spark feelings of gratitude.
- Be sure to also think about *why* you are grateful for each thing you list.
- Set a reminder on your phone or place your gratitude journal by your bed as a reminder.
- Keep the gratitude journal for as long as you like, a week, a month, a year. Some people keep gratitude diaries for decades.
- Sometimes it's hard, with chronic pain, to think about positives. If you find that's the case, ask a friend or loved one to help you count your blessings.

POSITIVE SERVICE

**DOMAINS: SOCIAL CONNECTIONS, POSITIVE EMOTIONS,
MEANING AND PURPOSE, PHYSICAL ACTIVITY**

Grateful people often pay it forward, which can land a powerful one-two punch that fights depressive symptoms. Paying it forward can come in the form of conducting kind acts for others, and one of the most meaningful kind acts is positive service. Volunteering your time to help a person or people, a community, or a cause is a positive service. Volunteering usually involves working through an organization and typically requires some level of sustained commitment ranging from a couple of hours to a year or more. You provide your time, talents, and skills for the good of the group. The reward comes in the form of satisfaction, gratitude, happiness, physical activity, and connection to the beneficiaries of the activities and other volunteers. If you're going to volunteer, do it with the mindset that your effort is helping others rather than yourself. But rest assured that you indeed will reap rich intangible rewards.

Try It Today

Engage in a volunteer activity. Many volunteer opportunities require planning, signing up in advance, or happen on specific days. Still, you can take the first steps today. Here are some ideas.

- Gather cans of food for a local food bank, drop them off, and ask the staff about volunteer opportunities.
- Donate gently worn clothes to a local charity shop, such as the Salvation Army or Goodwill, and ask them if they need volunteers.
- Talk to administrators at a community center, your place of worship, or your children's or grandchildren's school.
- Search volunteer opportunities in your community online. Most towns and cities have up-to-date opportunities for service.
- Lead a mini day of service and get a friend, neighbor, or family member to join you for a neighborhood park clean-up.

Make It Part of Your Thriving Plan

If you make positive service a pillar of your Thriving Plan, which I strongly encourage, here are some ideas for a more long-term commitment.

- Contact your local hospital, animal shelter, soup kitchen, public library, youth organization, parks department, or other organizations to learn more about volunteer opportunities.
- Here are a few more ideas: Volunteer at a hospital by reading to patients, playing music, or sharing your art; provide companionship for the elderly; knit hats for infants in the ICU; foster a shelter animal; register voters; tutor students; participate in clean-up days at local parks, forests, rivers, or lakes; organize a car wash to support a favorite charity; or coach a youth sports team.

DAY 27

APPRECIATE THE ARTS

DOMAINS: MEANING AND PURPOSE, POSITIVE EMOTIONS,

SOCIAL CONNECTIONS, PHYSICAL ACTIVITY

Beauty surrounds us. Today, I encourage you to open your eyes and mind to the remarkable talents of your fellow humans. Behind every beautiful painting, compelling dance performance, and soaring building, someone had a vision of creating something to cause you to weep, laugh, reflect, or even gasp. Think of today as a warm-up for experiencing awe, which we'll fully consider on Day 30. Let's spend today thinking about the visual and performing arts and harnessing their potential health benefits.

Try It Today

Consider what forms of the arts you can access today.

- Be open. If you have access to a museum of modern or contemporary art but don't like abstract art, try looking at the pieces with the fresh eyes of a child. I bet you can find one piece that speaks to you. Why do you like it?
- If you can attend a performance, then do that! Try to find something upbeat. While watching the performance, consider what feel-

ings spring up for you. Does it cause you to think? What emotions do you feel?

- Perhaps you have just enough time and energy to walk around town or your neighborhood. Consider the buildings. Think about the architects who designed them. Do the buildings have handsome details? Do they reflect a particular era?
- Do you have access to outdoor spaces with sculptures? Lots of cities and towns have public art or are creating public art spaces. If you're not sure, check online. If it's a nice day, pack a lunch or dinner and visit a public art space. Most of them have plenty of places to sit, and you also can watch the people looking at the art.
- If you can't get out today, click through a virtual exhibit of a favorite museum or somewhere you always have wanted to go. If you like dance, watch a performance of that on YouTube.

Make It Part of Your Thriving Plan

Adding the arts to your Thriving Plan can expand your activities, circle of friends, and positive emotions. Try to take a mini art outing once a week or every other week. Plan ahead so you can anticipate your adventure in the days leading up to it. If you have a visual impairment, more and more museums are offering tactile tours, or you can listen to audio plays and other adaptive experiences.

DAY 28

CULTIVATE PURPOSE IN LIFE

DOMAINS: MEANING AND PURPOSE, POSITIVE EMOTIONS

Remember, purpose *in* life differs from purpose *of* life, which we'll leave to philosophers and clerics. Instead, let's explore *your* specific purpose. For some people, life's purpose already appears clear. Almost without thinking, you might say that your purpose in life is to educate young children, care for the sick, raise healthy and productive kids, or cure heart disease. Most of us probably are thinking, *Um, where do I even start?* Well, today is all about taking that first step.

Try It Today

You don't find or discover purpose in life, like a four-leaf clover in a giant field of green. You cultivate it because it lies within you already! The way to know your purpose in life is to consider your values, passions, strengths, and abilities. Let's do a bit of that today.

- Clarify your values. Begin with identifying what you value most, such as parenthood, family, friends, romantic relationships, career, education, health and wellness, recreation or hobbies, community and service, equality and justice, and faith and spirituality. Also consider more concrete and more abstract entities, including nature, the environment, animals, personal growth, wisdom and learning, compassion, honor, financial success, the arts, leadership, inner peace, and world peace. There are no right or wrong answers—these are *your* values.

- What are your passions? What excites you? How do your passions map onto your values?

- What are your character strengths and how do these come into play? For example, if wisdom is a major character strength, does it complement your passion for, say, the arts? How might you be able to use your strengths to support your purpose?

- What are you good at already? Can you leverage your current knowledge, abilities, talents, and skills to help you lead a more purposeful life? How so?

- As you're thinking about these questions and ideas, jot down a few notes. For today, a good start is a good start! What are you considering for your purpose in life?

- Perhaps create a purpose-in-life statement. Here are some examples: "to feel accomplished in my career," "to educate and enrich the lives of young people," "to serve those who are less fortunate, "to remain constantly curious and searching for answers," "to be a spiritual, faithful, or enlightened person," and "to give my family love and support no matter what."

Make It Part of Your Thriving Plan

Purpose in life is a lifelong pursuit, but you can make evaluating your progress a regular occurrence, such as every New Year's Day or your birthday. To help guide you along the way, you might enjoy reading *Life on Purpose* by my colleague Vic Strecher at the University of Michigan. One more thought: Don't allow pain to dictate everything. Start with asking, "What would my life's purpose be if pain didn't figure into the equation?" Then go from there.

BEST POSSIBLE SELF

DOMAINS: MEANING AND PURPOSE, POSITIVE EMOTIONS

Visioning, or the practice of creating a positive mental picture of the future, can support your formulation or cultivation of purpose in life. The most effective visioning exercises involve imagining yourself happy, successful, and fulfilled at some point in the future. Seeing yourself succeed in a *realistic* pursuit and making that image as vivid as possible can help boost your mood now and help you chart a course toward that excellent prospect by identifying a series of small action steps to get you there.

Try It Today

- Gather pen and paper, a notebook or journal, or your computer or phone. Find a quiet and comfortable place where you can think and write for at least fifteen minutes.
- Pick a time in the future. It could be five or ten years from now or maybe just six months. Picture yourself in that point in time and imagine that everything has gone right. You may or may not still have pain, but you're *happy*. You are your best possible self.
- What has taken place to get you to that point? What specifically have you done or are in the process of doing? Is your health better than

expected because you started exercising and sleeping better? Are your relationships with family and friends (more) fulfilling? Have you found a greater sense of meaning and purpose in life?

- A caveat: Don't imagine yourself magically pain-free but do picture yourself better able to manage your pain. Any pain you might have has become far less bothersome.

- Don't picture unrealistic activities such as winning the Boston Marathon, performing on Broadway, or flying fighter jets—unless you already do or have done those activities—but do allow yourself to stretch your possibilities a bit.

- Spend the next couple of minutes visualizing how this future might look. Where might you be and with whom? How would you feel emotionally and physically?

- Engage your senses. What do you see, hear, smell, feel, and taste?

- Take the next ten minutes to write all these ideas down in as much detail as possible.

Make It Part of Your Thriving Plan

If you enjoy imagining your best possible self, spend a few minutes each day accessing this image of happiness and success and thinking about one very small, specific, achievable goal that you can set to help propel you toward realizing this goal. Let's say your desired future requires some additional training or classes. That's a big step. Possible smaller steps could include reading online about the topic, researching where such training or classes take place, learning about and comparing different options, evaluating costs in relation to your budget, discussing your plan with loved ones, talking with others who have similar training or do what you'd like to do, setting aside money to afford the first class, and finally enrolling. Learning how to break any large task or a series of tiny achievable goals (TAGs) is a great life skill for everyone!

TAKE AN "AWELIDAY"

**DOMAINS: MEANING AND PURPOSE, POSITIVE
EMOTIONS, SOCIAL CONNECTIONS**

Hooray! After traveling with me for the last twenty-nine days, I hope you're feeling a sense of accomplishment, hope, and anticipation. As we learned in Chapter 14, awe typically consists of feelings of positive self-diminishment and increased connectedness with other people. In a state of awe, we feel transcendence and focus less on ourselves and more on a meaningful whole. Awe doesn't require being religious. Anyone can feel a sense of awe when encountering the exceptional or superlative in nature, the arts, and human acts. For people with chronic pain, the part of the brain that processes rewarding experiences might need a little strength training and experiencing awe might be the perfect exercise. Remember, the areas of the brain that we regularly use tend to get stronger.

Try It Today

Awe tends to be spontaneous, but you can put yourself in situations more likely to inspire it. Today, we'll create a plan to help you find yourself in awe-inspiring moments in the future.

- List what you think might move you to a state of awe. Try to come up with five to ten ideas. A good way to think about this instruction is to answer the question: What wowed you in the past? If you're not sure, think about all the following possibilities.
- Spending time in nature. You can go someplace monumental, such as the Grand Canyon, Yellowstone, or Lake Michigan, or just a beautiful nearby park, farm, meadow, forest, or river.
- Attending a live performance. Go to a play, musical, concert, recital, dance performance, or other show that you're excited to experience.
- If you like sports, going to a sporting event for a game or team you love. Take in the history of the sport, the unity and pride of the crowd, the grandeur of the venue, and the talent of the athletes or players.
- Exploring an impressive architectural feat. Visit someplace amazing that you always have wanted to see, such as the Golden Gate Bridge, Statue of Liberty, Eiffel Tower, Burj Khalifa, or the Taj Mahal, or simply find a historic district near you and explore the history or details of the buildings.
- Attending a religious service or ceremony and immersing yourself in the experience. Breathe in the history, setting, community, words, music, and greater meaning.
- Order the activities that appeal to you noting the most achievable ones first. Pick what makes sense for your means and abilities and start to formulate a plan. If there's something you can do today, do it! Take a mini aweliday.

Make It Part of Your Thriving Plan

Plan and take regular awelidays, being mindful and present along the way. Experience each place or event with a sense of wonder as a child would and use all your senses. Lock in the moments by taking photos, journaling, or collecting souvenirs or mementos. Keep them in an "awebox" to preserve those moments of awe so you can revisit them and benefit from the feeling later.

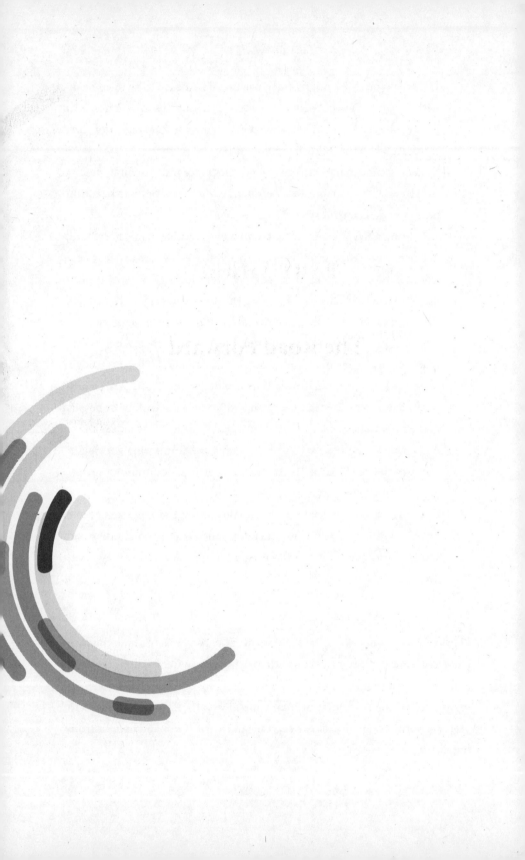

PART THREE

The Road Forward

CREATE YOUR THRIVING PLAN

Sometimes you must set aside deeply ingrained beliefs that are holding you back. Take chances, grab life by the throat, be daring, be persistent, and perhaps even feel a bit foolish. I'm asking you to do that and more, including making yourself a priority. This chapter will show you how to build your Thriving Plan, but first a quick story to illustrate that point.

We were traveling from Gainesville, Florida, to a national scientific meeting in Tampa. Kim Sibille—a close friend, excellent scientist, and lovely human being—was driving. In the distance, a large dark lump of debris was moving from the shoulder onto the highway.

"What's that?" she asked, squinting. We couldn't tell until we zoomed by.

"*Turtle!*" we both yelled.

"Should we do something?" Kim asked. The universe of what we could do seemed impossibly small. That turtle likely was going to be toast, but drivers and passengers also could be in danger.

"Sure?" I ventured.

She turned the car around using an access point in the center divider, and we returned to the turtle now halfway across the southbound lanes. The large hard-shelled turtle, probably 50 pounds, was lumbering along oblivious to the chaos it was creating. Cars were braking, honking, and swerving wildly. We pulled over into the breakdown lane and sprang into action. Kim threw open the trunk of her car and grabbed a pair of gloves and handed me a windshield wiper still in the box. I had no idea what purpose it could serve but took it anyway. We waded onto the highway, arms waving vigorously, hoping to be seen and to protect the turtle and other drivers. Cars stopped or cautiously crept around us. We bought the reptile enough time to make its way to the grassy center divider, halfway there. As we waited for it to cross the 25-yard stretch of wild grass, I had plenty of time to reflect. *What am I doing? This isn't me. I'm a rule follower. I do as expected, don't inconvenience anyone, and never break the law.* One stupid, dangerous act was demolishing all those conventions and we weren't done yet.

The turtle edged its way onto the northbound part of the highway, on which traffic was blessedly sparse. To my surprise, the windshield wiper made an incredibly effective turtle prod: *poke, poke, poke.* It reached halfway through the passing lane when the first wave of cars approached. They saw what we were doing, stopped, and put on their hazards. But another mass of cars and semis loomed in the distance, making the situation dire. In an act of inspiration, desperation, and madness, Kim donned the gloves, hoisted the turtle by its shell, and started carrying it to safety. Three steps into transport, it peed . . . a *lot.* Kim screamed, tossed her head back, and laughed but never dropped her charge. She made it to the other side of the highway. Traffic resumed, and the turtle ambled away into wild grassland. Sometimes we have to do things well outside our comfort zone: grab your life by the metaphorical shell, use everything you've got to lift it up, and carry it from the path of harm, pain, or suffering to reach a better place.

To recap: When stress, fear, resentment, hopelessness, anger, and sadness supercharge the pain circuits in our brain, the pain feels much worse. But mixing in joy, friendship, calm, love, purpose, and fun can influence the signals and make the pain better. That's the scientific premise for why and how a Thriving Plan could change your life for the better.

Most treatments for chronic pain don't work well for many people. If these medical interventions proved as effective as antibiotics for an infection or surgery for appendicitis, you likely wouldn't be reading this book. As someone who spends a lot of time conducting clinical trials in people with pain, I can tell you that many treatments fail or are only somewhat helpful if we study enough people. For what I mean by "somewhat," think of a drug where level-seven pain (on a scale of one to ten) declines to a five. You'd experience less pain, sure, but would that really constitute a life-changing treatment? Plus, what about all those pesky side effects?

Now, let me cheer you up a bit. In almost every treatment study for chronic pain, even those that fail to find evidence of effectiveness, some patients respond remarkably well. In a few of my studies, some patients recovered completely and returned to their normal lives, that small study of external qigong therapy for example. Perhaps we can attribute that improvement to the placebo effect but also perhaps not. For a considerable number of participants, the treatment is effective, whatever the underlying cause and whatever the treatment entails. Which raises the burning question: Who responds to what treatment, and how does that treatment work?

We're conducting two large studies to address those questions regarding seven common treatments for people with chronic low back pain as part of the HEAL initiative Back Pain Consortium (HEAL BACPAC) funded by the National Institutes of Health. While we await the results of those and similar studies, the pain field continues moving toward embracing patient preferences and individualized treatments. (*Hooray!*) New clinical trials often have more complicated designs taking into consideration that treatment needs flexibility—including tailoring to an individual patient's needs, combining two or more treatments, and acceptability—meaning the treatment must make sense to patients and be something that they're willing to do.

Your Thriving Plan rests firmly on all those ideas: it's personalized, flexible, and based on what makes sense to you and, hopefully, what you're willing to do. The last point is perhaps most critical. One way that Western medicine often fails people with chronic pain is that most treatments involve something done *to* a patient and usually just once. I'm proposing the opposite. You select the elements that will form the foundation for a radical shift in your life for the better. You create a plan that's unique to you, makes sense to you, and to which you commit yourself over time.

Living your Thriving Plan might feel foreign or artificial at first, and that's OK. After some time, the skills you develop and retain will become habits. You may not remember anymore, but, when you were a kid, brushing your teeth felt weird at first, too, but the skill became a healthy daily habit. Same idea!

What Goes into a Thriving Plan?

Your Thriving Plan might work best if a few of the larger principles from the earlier chapters of the book guide it, namely understanding that:

- The brain amplifies pain and can generate it completely on its own (top-down pain). Many of the seemingly unrelated activities that you tried in the thirty-day exploration period eventually can influence changes in the brain that will result in less pain.
- Thoughts, emotions, and behaviors such as exercise, sleep, and socializing increase or decrease pain signals. You have the power to influence how your brain processes pain by changing your thoughts, emotions, and behavior.
- Skills and techniques that promote healthy self-esteem, positive emotions, self-compassion, helpful actions (get moving and sleep better), and healthy relationships work as the cornerstones of resilience, setting the stage for less pain and better overall health.

To address these important principles, your Thriving Plan needs to have multiple facets. In other words, you'll choose activities and goals that address several domains in your life. Following are the key domains and some related activities, skills, and practices.

RELAXATION	Calm down, unwind, and destress. These activities could include a breathing practice, meditation, progressive muscle relaxation, guided imagery, engaging in a hobby, music, and more.
BETTER SLEEP	If you sleep poorly, this is a great place to start! Try relaxation skills along with developing better sleep habits, such as going to bed and waking up at the same time every day.
ADAPTIVE THOUGHTS	Think more optimistic thoughts with at least four approaches to consider. Pick one to start and see how this new way of thinking resonates over time. Try another after that if you like.
PHYSICAL ACTIVITY	Get moving with a walking program, swimming, biking, dancing, yoga, or doing other daily activities with more oomph. Try activity pacing and scheduling pleasant activities to support your success.
POSITIVE EMOTIONS	Make room for more joy, contentment, and fun. This domain might seem frivolous, but it could be the most important. Consider practicing gratitude, savoring, keeping a positive piggy bank, listening to your favorite music, or spending time in nature.
SOCIAL CONNECTIONS	Cultivate rewarding relationships that will build your relationship tree. These activities include making daily connections, doing kind acts, practicing forgiveness, and giving of your time and your heart.
MEANING & PURPOSE	Focus on your values and living a life filled with meaning. Positive service, cultivating your unique purpose in life, envisioning your best possible self, and being open to awe all can inspire hope even on the darkest days.

You'll notice that none of the domains are "Improve Pain" because *all the domains and related activities can help improve your pain and ability to function.*

Creating the Plan

Begin with tools that feel most comfortable to you: pen and paper, personal journal, computer, or the Thriving Plan worksheet that you can find at the end of this chapter or downloadable at AftonHassett.com (Resources). Go back through the thirty activities, practices, and skills (let's refer to them as "activities" for now) and identify the activities you *really* liked. Look for the stars! For each activity that you starred, make a note of every domain that it touches. Many of the activities involve multiple domains, but the first domain listed is primary, and the rest are secondary. Ideally, you want have to a couple of activities in each domain.

Next, you need to make some decisions about what activities you want in your plan for what purpose. To get started, look at your list and identify the most exciting activity in each domain. After that, prioritize the domains by ranking them from one to seven with one representing the top priority. Then, decide whether you want a given activity to address multiple domains or a specific activity for each domain. For example, let's say that Pleasant Activity Scheduling is something you're excited to do because your chosen pleasant activity to schedule is Pickleball. This is awesome because Pickleball is great for physical exercise and it's a social activity, too. In this case, one activity covers two domains: Physical Activity and Social Connections.

You'll want to try some of these activities over time before committing to them, so you might have a Plan A and a Plan B in each domain. You also can do something for a while, tire of it, and give it up. Perhaps you already have a good habit for one of the domains and want to add something new to it, which would be great! However you want to plan and arrange it is the best way to do it because it's *your* plan. It should make sense to you and feel exciting. I've included an example of a Thriving Plan worksheet here, but you might organize your own plan totally differently to suit your needs and preferences.

Sample Worksheet

DOMAIN	PRIMARY	SECONDARY	MOST EXCITING	PRIORITY
RELAXATION	Paced breathing PMR Nature breaks	Music is medicine Healthy sleep habits	Nature breaks Paced breathing	2
BETTER SLEEP	Healthy sleep habits	Paced breathing Walking program PMR		1
ADAPTIVE THOUGHTS	Reframing Coping coach Self-compassion	Positive piggy bank Gratitude diary	Reframing	3
PHYSICAL ACTIVITY	Walking program Positive service	Pleasant activity scheduling Nature breaks	Walking program	4
POSITIVE EMOTIONS	Positive piggy bank Music is medicine Pleasant activity scheduling	Nature breaks Self-compassion Positive service Plan an aweliday	Music is medicine	5
SOCIAL CONNECTIONS	Daily connection Positive service	Walking program Pleasant activity scheduling Planning an aweliday	Positive service	7
MEANING & PURPOSE	Gratitude diary Planning an aweliday	Pleasant activity Nature breaks Positive piggy bank Music is medicine Positive service	Planning an aweliday	6

In this sample, sleep ranks as the top priority, but other practices and skills are more exciting. That's fine. Perhaps this person will start by working on unhelpful sleep practices while practicing a more exciting activity from the Relaxation domain (second top priority), such as mastering paced breathing or taking daily nature breaks. If this person is feeling ambitious, a walking program would overlap nicely with improving sleep, social connections, and those fun nature breaks. For most people, trying three new activities at once would be too much! A couple of weeks down the road, it might be nice to try pleasant activity scheduling for a few weeks—because it covers a few domains—and see how that goes. Further down the road: reframing, keeping a positive piggy bank, or planning an "aweliday" as a reward for all this hard work. There's no single way to do this; it's up to you. Maybe pull out those highlighters to see what activities appear most often. In the example, Positive Service comes up in four domains. Remember, you can also do just one activity at a time for as long as you like and add one or more new activities whenever you are ready. The final chapter contains essential tips and suggestions for organizing and living your Thriving Plan now and for the long run. Please don't skip it! But for today, I encourage you to spend some time setting the foundation for your Thriving Plan and get ready to begin a new phase of your life.

Your Thriving Plan Worksheet

DOMAIN	PRIMARY	SECONDARY	MOST EXCITING	PRIORITY
RELAXATION				
BETTER SLEEP				
ADAPTIVE THOUGHTS				
PHYSICAL ACTIVITY				
POSITIVE EMOTIONS				
SOCIAL CONNECTIONS				
MEANING & PURPOSE				

Notes

_____

_____

_____

_____

_____

_____

_____

_____

_____

_____

_____

_____

_____

_____

_____

_____

Lived Experience: Lynne

Years ago, I moved to a new city. To make friends, I joined a group of women who met once a week to share and support one another. The first time I attended, all I could see were "perfect" women. They dressed beautifully, spoke eloquently, and had successful careers. It became clear that I had to be as "perfect" as they were. I worked hard to dress perfectly, went above and beyond to give nice gifts, and planned perfect events. But it still felt like it wasn't enough. When I learned they were having a party and didn't invite me, it was devastating. I had tried so hard to fit in.

A few days after the party, I mustered the courage to ask one of the women, Carol, why I wasn't invited. I couldn't hold back the tears, which shocked Carol.

"Why are you crying?" she said softly.

I was so embarrassed. I wanted to run away, but I had shown my vulnerability, so I told her what I was feeling. I explained that I had tried to be perfect for the group, spending money I didn't have on clothes and going to the salon they all went to, and I didn't know what I had done wrong.

"You have it all wrong!" Carol replied. "The reason you weren't invited was because it was a T-shirt and sweatpants party. We didn't think you'd want to go. In fact, some people in the group have commented that *you* probably think that *we* aren't good enough for you."

I couldn't believe it! How could they think that I wouldn't go to a casual party and that I thought I was better than them? They totally misinterpreted all my efforts. I had tried so hard, and they didn't understand. For days, I thought about my life and relationships. I thought about what Carol had told me, realizing that they had seen me as a different person because I hadn't been myself. Being a perfectionist wasn't producing good results. I would never be perfect, and it was better to live my life in a healthier way and to give up trying to reach the unattainable.

I asked Carol and the other women to meet me for coffee. The next day, in an old running outfit, I jogged to the coffee shop and arrived sweaty.

I told them I was struggling to fit into my new community and asked if they'd help me get to know the area better. Carol immediately suggested that they all go for a run around town every Tuesday and asked if I would like to join. I enthusiastically accepted the invitation, and immediately a huge weight lifted off me. I was letting go of perfectionism, and life seemed better already.

Trying to be "perfect" or live the life of a perfectionist is not only futile but also causes many negative effects. Perfectionism can disrupt your relationships, make it impossible to accomplish tasks or goals, and, by setting unachievable expectations, you will feel insecure, overwhelmed, and unsatisfied. The belief that you must be perfect can stop you even from trying. So let go of perfectionism, put on your sweatpants, ruffle up your hair, and give it a try.

———

Lynne Kennedy Matallana is president of Community Health Focus, Inc., and PainTools, its self-care program.

LIVE YOUR THRIVING PLAN

OK, you have started the process of formulating a Thriving Plan that hopefully excites you. Yippee! Well, what now? Let's think about the next phase of your life as a grand experiment. Your Thriving Plan is a living document. Try activities, practice them, adopt them, or reject them, then move on to other ones, always keeping what you like and what works and letting go of the rest. That's pretty much how scientists do research. We have an idea about what might work, we test the idea, and, depending on that outcome, we retain, modify, or reject the idea and then proceed to the next indicated step. Even though we initially thought we had *the* answer, we try not to hold onto what doesn't work. We must remain open to where the data take us.

That means that you need to be open to failure. That's right; you and your Thriving Plan *don't need to be perfect!* Perfectionism is unusually common in people with chronic pain. It's not clear why, but if that sounds like you, you're not alone. The problem with perfectionism, especially if self-critical, is that it could undermine your success. So, especially if you're a perfectionist, embrace your imperfections! You know what they are. Be willing to try something new and maybe a little bit ruffled and messy.

Where to Begin?

Your Thriving Plan addresses seven domains, and you probably have identified two or more activities for each domain. The numbers can feel overwhelming, but you shouldn't do everything all at once. It's a long-term plan executed in stages and subject to change, just like real life. Focus on one or two activities total for a few weeks or a month. Consider starting with the activity that seems the most fun, rewarding, or motivating or the one that primarily addresses your most important domain.

Remember, back in Chapter 2, when we considered SPACE? Sleep, Pain, Affect (emotions), Cognition (concentration, memory, clarity), and Energy—some or all of these symptoms tend to occur in people with chronic pain. Poor sleep and mood often aggravate pain, brain fog, and low energy. If you have bouts of insomnia or rarely feel refreshed when you wake, start with activities in the Relaxation and Sleep domains. In the context of treating chronic pain, fixing sleep counts as low-hanging fruit. If you sleep better, a lot of other symptoms generally will improve, including your pain. If you sleep well but have anxiety, depression, or just feel emotionally blah, dive into Positive Emotions and Adaptive Thoughts to start.

If you don't have either of those difficulties, let's get you moving! The Physical Activity domain represents an excellent start for everyone. If you feel lonely, need support, or have difficult relationships, prioritize activities in the Social Connections domain. The domain of Meaning and Purpose appears at the bottom of the list and in later chapters because it's a higher-order need. Attend to your survival needs first: sleep; get moving; feel happier, more hopeful, and then supported by friends and family. Now, revisit the priority list on your Thriving Plan worksheet, did you have it right in the context of your SPACE symptoms? Next, circle the one or maybe two domains that you will focus on first and pick one related skill, ideally something you are excited about.

Set Tiny Achievable Goals

Now that you know where you want to start, set tiny achievable goals (TAGs). Specificity and a reasonable time limit will make them achievable. Let's use a goal in the domain of Physical Activity for an example: say that you want to walk briskly with hand weights for thirty minutes five days per week. That's an outstanding goal, but you can't get there right away. A good first TAG could be walking briskly for five minutes three days a week. If you haven't walked briskly in a while, those five minutes will feel like a worthy and hopefully achievable goal. Your next TAG could be walking briskly for ten minutes four days a week, then fifteen minutes five days per week. It's OK to adjust big goals because achieving a smaller goal that sticks matters more than having an overly ambitious goal that falls by the wayside.

Hitting big goals requires hitting lots of tiny goals first. Marathoners don't just assemble at the starting line and complete the race. They put in months of incremental training, achieving scores of personal goals along the way. Don't hold yourself to a different standard. Build up to big goals with lots of tiny ones. Here's a critical related idea: Little changes that last are better than big changes lost over time. Nothing is too small. Even repeating a goal matters because it means you've got the grit to achieve it more than once, which is great! Any improvement is excellent improvement, and it all adds up. If you walk just twenty more steps per day, every day, you'll be walking an additional 7,300 steps per day by the end of a year. That's more than three miles!

Set Reminders so You Can Remember to Remember

You know what I mean. The whole system breaks down if you simply forget to do what you need to do. Once you set big goals and the TAGs to get you there, decide how you want to remind yourself. Put activities on your calendar, sticky notes on the fridge, or reminders in your phone. Reminders can have more nuance or meaning to them, too. A vase of flowers on the counter = garden today. If you need a little more encouragement, buddy up with a friend who will do the activity with you. Also try setting a reward for completing the committed activity. Maybe tack a picture of that reward on your bathroom mirror or make it the home screen on your phone or computer.

Give It Time to Work

As discussed right before you began the thirty-day exploration period, no one is likely to generate immediate results. The goal of the thirty-day period was to figure out what makes sense to you and what you will want to try and repeat later. A proper try, that I'd like you to do as part of your Thriving Plan, consists of doing the activity regularly, possibly daily, for at least two weeks. If, at the end of two weeks, you like a particular activity and it seems helpful, make it a habit. Practicing the activities makes them skills, and repeating the skills makes them habits.

Track Your Progress

You might want to start with a symptom log. You can find a great symptom tracker at PainGuide.com. With it, you can log one, two, or even all the SPACE symptoms daily, which can be incredibly informative when judging whether an activity is helping. Once we feel better, sometimes we forget just how bad our pain felt, and we may not realize how changes positively impact symptoms and the ability to function.

You also could use an activity tracker, such as a Fitbit, which makes it easier to track physical activity and sleep. This type of tracking could help you identify hidden improvement, too. What does hidden improvement mean? Well, in clinical trials, we've found that sometimes, when we use only pain as the measure of response to treatment, we might miss the effect of a particular therapy. When someone starts a treatment study, a person might say his or her pain is a five and then, at the end of the study, a four. A one-point change doesn't seem like much benefit, but we have learned that, if you talk to that person, he or she might be feeling *so much better* and doing many more and more meaningful activities than before, creating a happier and richer life. Even slight improvement allows people to do more and make up for lost time. That increased activity can leave pain levels a little high, but study participants made that choice for themselves, and they're good with it! When you track your progress, remember that the same effect could be happening in your life, too.

Tips for Establishing New Habits

Many theories touch on how best to establish new habits and ditch bad ones that no longer serve you. My favorite approaches are gloriously simple. The best? Make the new habit you want to form something you really want to do. We're wired to do what brings us pleasure and avoid what causes us pain. That's why, when establishing your Thriving Plan, make the first new habit you want to form something that excites you or seems fun to do. So, to address the domain of Physical Activity, don't pick an exercise that feels overly ambitious or like drudgery. If you love to dance, find a dance-oriented exercise class or maybe take ballroom dancing.

In *Good Habits, Bad Habits: The Science of Making Positive Changes That Stick*, researcher and psychologist Wendy Wood at the University of Southern California notes that almost half of our daily behaviors consist of habits. These automatic activities require little conscious thought. We just do them. She suggests that willpower and motivation might start us down the right path, but they're not enough to make a habit stick. Instead, we need to make the new habit easy to do and then reward ourselves when we do it. Let's say you want to begin your day with paced breathing. First, make it easy to do by setting your alarm several minutes early, putting an eye-catching reminder next to your bed, and promising yourself a little reward for completing your breathing practice as planned.

In *Habit Stacking: 97 Small Life Changes That Take Five Minutes or Less*, Steve Scott developed another approach. Habit stacking involves identifying already established habits and adding a new activity to them. For example, if you brush your teeth after breakfast and before bed and you want to make a habit of stretching twice a day, how about stretching right after brushing your teeth? Another example might be if you have the habit of checking your email first thing every morning, and the new habit you want to form is reaching out to one person daily to build your social connections, then how about sending that friendly email out then? Making a list of people to email and setting a reminder or leaving a visual cue can help the process until this new stacked habit becomes, well, a habit.

New Habits Take Time

At the CPFRC, my colleague and friend Dave Williams has a great analogy for explaining how habits take hold and work. Imagine the landscape of your life as a big open prairie that no one has crossed. The first wagon that passes over the land bumps along, weaving to and fro. The next wagon follows that first path, but maybe smooths the way a bit. Wagon after wagon follows that path, the wheel grooves becoming obvious and deep, forming a safe, reliable track. Habits behave a lot like that. A new habit you're trying to form feels uncomfortable, and you may not execute it perfectly. Over time, it streamlines, becoming more ingrained, and then simply becomes what you do without a lot of thought.

Get Others Onboard

Many obstacles and people will get in the way of you taking care of yourself—but only if you allow it. Follow in the footsteps of Michelle Andwele, who called on you to start a new chapter in your life called "Priority: Me" on page 149. Remember, if you don't take care of yourself, you can't take care of anyone else. Of course, you still should make time in your day and space in your heart for the people you love but strike a balance between attending to everyone else and attending to yourself.

To rally the support you need, let others know that you're going on this journey. Include them in the adventure where it makes sense and where they might feel some excitement. At the very least, let them know how important this reset is to you and ask for their support and encouragement. Then perhaps plan regular outings with friends, a walking program with a family member, or an aweliday with your significant other.

Words of Wisdom: Patience, Flexibility, and Self-Compassion

Pain psychologist, fellow researcher, and friend Lindsey McKernan at Vanderbilt University shared three more points for you to consider as you work on your Thriving Plan. First, she suggests that, when establishing new goals, it helps to distinguish between a realistic starting point and where you ideally want to be. The disconnect between those two different places can cause a lot of internal turmoil because you might feel embarrassed or ashamed about where you are at the present moment and where you want to be can seem impossibly far away. These thoughts and feelings are normal, and TAGs can help you move closer to your bigger goals every single day.

Second, be flexible and know that capturing the essence of an activity that you used to love can make an excellent stepping stone. You may not be able to participate fully in the activity in the same way that you once did, but you still can bring meaning and value to it. For example, if you love tennis and can't play anymore, you still can attend events, coach a team, or gently volley the ball back and forth with an understanding friend. Being too hard on yourself risks losing out on these fun, fulfilling activities as a result.

Lastly, beware of that nasty internal critic. (Remember our discussion of chatter in Chapter 4?) If you tend to self-criticize or negatively evaluate changes or experiences while attempting to reach your goals, re-envision challenging moments or setbacks as normal and an opportunity for self-compassion. Accept that change is difficult but worth it. Remember, self-compassion is simply giving yourself the same understanding and encouragement that you would give a dear friend.

Final Thoughts

We've covered a lot of ground! By now, I hope you feel informed, energized, and ready to begin the next phase of your life. You've met some amazing people, including several of my colleagues and others who have lived experiences perhaps like your own. I hope what you have learned about your brain has laid the groundwork for you to have a meaningful relationship with the conductor of your symphony. As you know, you will have good days and bad. I hope you go into each armed with the knowledge that this is a process. Like the stock market, you're investing for the future, so plan on weathering the ups and downs. On bad days, just do one activity that's meaningful or that makes you happy. No matter how lousy you feel or how bad the day, you'll have experienced something positive, which means that lousy day still matters.

I wish for you a life filled with family and friends, memorable adventures as well as quiet moments of reflection, lots of laughter and love, and a caring relationship with yourself and your brain. Thank you for the gift of your time.

ACKNOWLEDGMENTS

THERE ARE SO MANY PEOPLE TO THANK, and I'm certain that I'll forget some of my favorites. Sorry! Please let me know, and I'll treat you to lunch and an acknowledgment in my next book, if I'm lucky enough to earn that honor.

Let's start with my beloved husband, Will, my biggest cheerleader, who does everything possible to help me flourish—from grocery shopping to handling the complex business aspects of writing. Thank you. I'd be lost without you, I love you all there is. To my stepson, Liam, who sees me as the person I want to be. I am so proud of the renaissance man you have become, your service to our country, and my mighty fine grand-dog, Jefe. Liam, I always will do my best so that you'll be proud of me, too.

A shout-out to three people whose contributions made this book possible. First, a big-time thank you to Steve Pierce, the talented illustrator who has helped translate my crazy ideas into beautiful art. You breathe life into pen and ink. Second, to Stacey Glick, the only agent whom Will and I wanted because we knew on some cosmic level that you were the right one. Stacey, you had us at the Mets. To James Jayo, my exceptional editor, and the entire crew at Countryman Press, thank you for giving this new author a shot and for having the good sense to steer me in the right direction.

As a scientist, I fussed endlessly about how to share complex scientific concepts precisely and understandably. To do this with any success, I had to lean on the goodwill of my colleagues and friends. Thank you to Dan

Clauw, not only for being supportive and helping me think through key chapters but also for your friendship and for giving me the opportunity to be a part of this incomparable research team. You have built something special at the Chronic Pain and Fatigue Reaserch Center, and your kindness and generosity embody the beloved University of Michigan mantra, "The Team, the Team, the Team." Dave Williams, I'm grateful for your helpful insights and suggestions for this book, but more importantly thanks for all the years of comradery, mentorship, and laughter.

Other content experts, a blanket thank-you to the neuroscience squad: Steve Harte, Rick Harris, Chelsea Kaplan, and Andrew Schrepf. Your knowledge of the human brain never ceases to amaze. Your knowledge of the heart makes all of you great scientists and friends.

A special group hug to my fellow clinical psychologists, some of whom appear in this book: Lindsey McKernan, Kim Sibille, Tony King, Jenna McAfee, Anna Kratz, Drew Sturgeon, and Dave Williams (again). Your insights and suggestions related to your specialty areas, behavior change more broadly, and how to help readers get the most from this book were invaluable.

My gratitude also goes to Jen Pierce, a social psychologist, who helped me think and talk about the devastating effects of trauma in people with pain, as well as the sublime power of our social connections for recovery. Three cheers to Kevin Boehnke, who gave me wise counsel about the art of writing and who generously shared his lived experience. A special thank you to the ever-cheeky Daniel Whibley, a physiotherapist who studies sleep and pain. Your help with the exercise and sleep chapters is appreciated, as was the boost of confidence you gave me when I most needed it.

Thank you, Chad Brummett, for building the critical research infrastructure at the Back & Pain Center and then entrusting me with the keys. The work you do has radically changed the practice of medicine for the better. I am also grateful for our incomparable leaders at the departmental level, first Dr. Tremper (who will always be *Dr.* Temper) and now George Mashour. Both of your support for this pain psychologist who studies unconventional topics has always been felt and deeply appreciated.

My acknowledgments would be incomplete without recognition of my early career mentors Marian Stuart, Robert Pinals, and especially Len Sigal. Without your support and advocacy in those early years, I wouldn't have had this remarkable experience. I think about your generosity and wise counsel often and hope to provide similar insightful and supportive mentorship to my FIERCE mentees.

Lastly, my deepest gratitude to the people with lived experience who bravely shared their stories in this book, as well as those whom I have met in therapy sessions, casual conversations on airplanes, the bustling halls at scientific meetings, and really everywhere. Your courage inspires me, and your hope fuels me.

NOTES

1   Mary-Ann Fitzcharles et al., "Nociplastic Pain: Towards an Understanding of Preva-
    lent Pain Conditions," *Lancet* 397, no. 10289 (May 29, 2021): 2098–110; Michael C,
    Lee and Irene Tracey, "Unravelling the Mystery of Pain, Suffering, and Relief with
    Brain Imaging," *Current Pain and Headache Reports* 14, no. 2 (April 2010):124–31;
    Vitaly Napadow and Richard E. Harris, "What Has Functional Connectivity and
    Chemical Neuroimaging in Fibromyalgia Taught Us About the Mechanisms and Man-
    agement of 'Centralized' Pain?" *Arthritis Research & Therapy* 16, no. 5 (2014): 425.
2   Chelsea M. Kaplan et al., "Functional and Neurochemical Disruptions of Brain Hub
    Topology in Chronic Pain," *Pain* 160, no. 4 (April 2019): 973–83.
3   Andrew Schrepf et al., "Sensory Sensitivity and Symptom Severity Represent Unique
    Dimensions of Chronic Pain: A MAPP Research Network Study," *Pain* 159, no. 10
    (October 2018):2002–11.
4   Richard H. Gracely et al., "Functional Magnetic Resonance Imaging Evidence of
    Augmented Pain Processing in Fibromyalgia," *Arthritis & Rheumatism* 46 no. 5 (May
    2002): 1333–43; Thorsten Giesecke et al., "Evidence of Augmented Central Pain
    Processing in Idiopathic Chronic Low Back Pain," *Arthritis & Rheumatism* 50, no.
    2 (February 2004): 613–23; Jason J. Kutch et al., "Brain Signature and Functional
    Impact of Centralized Pain: A Multidisciplinary Approach to the Study of Chronic
    Pelvic Pain (MAPP) Network Study," *Pain* 158, no. 10 (October 2017): 1979–91;
    Adriane Icenhour et al., "Brain Functional Connectivity Is Associated with Vis-
    ceral Sensitivity in Women with Irritable Bowel Syndrome," *NeuroImage Clinical* 15
    (June 2, 2017): 449–57; Jesus Pujol et al., "Brain Imaging of Pain Sensitization in
    Patients with Knee Osteoarthritis," *Pain* 158, no. 9 (September 2017):1831–38; Todd
    J. Schwedt et al., "Allodynia and Descending Pain Modulation in Migraine: A Rest-
    ing State Functional Connectivity Analysis," *Pain Medicine* 15, no. 1 (January 2014):
    154–65; Jarred W. Younger et al., "Chronic Myofascial Temporomandibular Pain Is

Associated with Neural Abnormalities in the Trigeminal and Limbic Systems," *Pain* 149, no. 2 (May 2010): 222–28.

5 Mary-Ann Fitzcharles et al., "Nociplastic Pain: Towards an Understanding of Prevalent Pain Conditions," *Lancet* 397, no. 10289 (May 29, 2021): 2098–110.

6 Dillon J. Newbold et al., "Plasticity and Spontaneous Activity Pulses in Disused Human Brain Circuits," *Neuron* 107, no. 3 (August 5, 2020): 580–89.

7 Andrew Schrepf et al., "Top Down or Bottom Up? An Observational Investigation of Improvement in Fibromyalgia Symptoms Following Hip and Knee Replacement," *Rheumatology (Oxford)* 59, no. 3 (March 1, 2020): 594–602.

8 Daniel J. Clauw, "Fibromyalgia: A Clinical Review," *The Journal of the American Medical Association* 311, no. 15 (April 16, 2014): 1547–55; Mary-Ann Fitzcharles et al., "Nociplastic Pain: Towards an Understanding of Prevalent Pain Conditions," *Lancet* 397, no. 10289 (May 29, 2021): 2098–110; Tony E. Larkin et al., "Altered Network Architecture of Functional Brain Communities in Chronic Nociplastic Pain," *NeuroImage* 226 (February 1, 2021): 117504; Steven E. Harte et al., "Pharmacologic Attenuation of Cross-Modal Sensory Augmentation within the Chronic Pain Insula," *Pain* 157, no. 9 (September 2016): 1933–45; Richard E. Harris et al., "Decreased Central μ-Opioid Receptor Availability in Fibromyalgia," *Journal of Neuroscience* 27, no. 37 (September 12, 2007): 10000–6.

9 Francois Lesperance, Nancy Frasure-Smith, and Mario Talajic, "Major Depression Before and After Myocardial Infarction: Its Nature and Consequences," *Psychosomatic Medicine* 58, no. 2 (March–April 1996): 99–110; Christopher M Celano and Jeff C Huffman, "Depression and Cardiac Disease: A Review," *Cardiology in Review* 19, no. 3 (May–June 2011): 130–42.

10 Chelsea M. Kaplan et al., "Neurobiological Antecedents of Multisite Pain in Children," *Pain* 163, no. 4 (April 1, 2022): e596–e603; Chelsea Kaplan, et al., "Risk Factors for the Development of Multisite Pain in Children," under review at *The Clinical Journal of Pain*.

11 I researched and wrote this case in collaboration with Dr. Robert Pinals, one of my most beloved mentors and the Obi-Wan Kenobi of rheumatology. Thanks, Bob! Robert S. Pinals and Afton L. Hassett, "Reconceptualizing John F. Kennedy's Chronic Low Back Pain," *Regional Anesthesia & Pain Medicine* 38, no. 5 (September–October 2013): 442–6.

12 Andrew Schrepf et al., "Sensory Sensitivity and Symptom Severity Represent Unique Dimensions of Chronic Pain: A MAPP Research Network Study," *Pain* 159, no. 10 (October 2018):2002–11.

13 Elizabeth D. Hale, Diane C. Radvanski, and Afton L. Hassett, "The Man-in-the-Moon Face: A Qualitative Study of Body Image, Self-Image and Medication Use in Systemic Lupus Erythematosus," *Rheumatology (Oxford)* 54, no. 7 (July 2015): 1220–25.

14 Afton L. Hassett and Daniel J. Clauw "Does Psychological Stress Cause Chronic Pain?" *Psychiatric Clinics of North America* 34, no. 3 (September 2011): 579–94; Afton L. Hassett and Daniel J. Clauw, "The Role of Stress in Rheumatic Diseases," *Arthritis Research & Therapy* 12, no. 3 (2010): 123.

15 Lesley M. Arnold et al., "Family Study of Fibromyalgia," *Arthritis & Rheumatism* 50, no. 3 (March 2004): 944–52.

16 Gary D. Slade et al., "Painful Temporomandibular Disorder: Decade of Discovery from OPPERA Studies," *Journal of Dental Research* 95, no. 10 (September 2016): 1084–92; Samuel A. McLean et al. "Catechol *O*-Methyltransferase Haplotype Predicts Immediate Musculoskeletal Neck Pain and Psychological Symptoms After Motor Vehicle Collision," *The Journal of Pain* 12, no. 1 (January 2011): 101–7; Jacob N. Ablin and Dan Buskila, "Update on the Genetics of the Fibromyalgia Syndrome," *Best Practice & Research Clinical Rheumatology* 29, no. 1 (February 2015): 20–8.

17 Daniel J. Clauw et al., "Considering the Potential for an Increase in Chronic Pain After the COVID-19 Pandemic," *Pain* 161, no. 8 (August 2020): 1694–97.

18 Robert Dantzer et al., "Cytokines and Sickness Behavior," *Annals of the New York Academy of Sciences* 840 (May 1, 1998): 586–90.

19 Bruce S. McEwen and Elizabeth N. Lasley, *The End of Stress As We Know It* (Washington, DC: Joseph Henry Press, 2002).

20 Asmina Lazaridou et al., "Effects of Cognitive-Behavioral Therapy (CBT) on Brain Connectivity Supporting Catastrophizing in Fibromyalgia," *The Clinical Journal of Pain* 33, no. 3 (March 2017): 215–21.

21 Ethan Kross, *Chatter: The Voice in Our Head, Why It Matters, and How to Harness It* (New York: Crown, 2021).

22 Attila Galambos et al., "A Systematic Review of Structural and Functional MRI Studies on Pain Catastrophizing," *Journal of Pain Research* 12 (April 11, 2019): 1155–78; Richard H. Gracely et al., "Pain Catastrophizing and Neural Responses to Pain Among Persons with Fibromyalgia," *Brain* 127, no. 4 (April 2004): 835–43.

23 Afton L. Hassett et al., "Association Between Predeployment Optimism and Onset of Postdeployment Pain in US Army Soldiers," *JAMA Network Open* 2, no. 2 (February 1, 2019): e188076.

24 Felix Brandl et al., "Common and Specific Large-Scale Brain Changes in Major Depressive Disorder, Anxiety Disorders, and Chronic Pain: A Transdiagnostic Multimodal Meta-Analysis of Structural and Functional MRI Studies," *Neuropsychopharmacololgy* 47 (2022): 1071–80.

25 Daniel Goleman, *Emotional Intelligence: Why It Can Matter More Than IQ* (New York: Bantam Books, 1995).

26 Afton L. Hassett et al., "Affect and Low Back Pain: More to Consider Than the Influence of Negative Affect Alone," *The Clinical Journal of Pain* 32, no. 10 (October 2016): 907–14; Loren L. Toussaint et al., "A Comparison of Fibromyalgia Symptoms in Patients with Healthy versus Depressive, Low and Reactive Affect Balance Styles," *Scandinavian Journal of Pain* 5, no. 3 (March 1, 2014): 161–66; Afton L. Hassett and Patrick H. Finan, "The Role of Resilience in the Clinical Management of Chronic Pain," *Current Pain and Headache Reports* 20, no. 6 (June 2016): 39; Afton L. Hassett et al., "The Relationship Between Affect Balance Style and Clinical Outcomes in Fibromyalgia," *Arthritis Care & Research* 59, no. 6 (June 15, 2008): 833–40.

27 Barbara L. Fredrickson, "The Broaden-and-Build Theory of Positive Emotions," *Philosophical Transactions of the Royal Society of London B: Biological Sciences* 359, no. 1449 (September 20, 2004): 1367–78.

28 Rebecca Alexander et al., "The Neuroscience of Positive Emotions and Affect: Implications for Cultivating Happiness and Wellbeing," *Neuroscience and Biobehavioral Reviews* 121 (February 2021): 220–49.

29 Eric L. Garland, Brett Froeliger, and Matthew O. Howard, "Effects of Mindfulness-Oriented Recovery Enhancement on Reward Responsiveness and Opioid Cue-Reactivity," *Psychopharmacology* 231, no. 16 (August 2014): 3229–38; Sasha Gorrell, Megan E. Shott, and Guido K.W. Frank, "Associations Between Aerobic Exercise and Dopamine-Related Reward-Processing: Informing a Model of Human Exercise Engagement," *Biological Psychology* 171 (May 2022): 108350; Maria Kryza-Lacombe et al., "Changes in Neural Reward Processing Following Amplification of Positivity Treatment for Depression and Anxiety: Preliminary Findings from a Randomized Waitlist Controlled Trial," *Behaviour Research & Therapy* 142 (July 2021): 103860.

30 Niloofar Afari et al., "Psychological Trauma and Functional Somatic Syndromes: A Systematic Review and Meta-Analysis," *Psychosomatic Medicine* 76, no. 1 (January 2014): 2–11; Robert R. Edwards et al., "The Role of Psychosocial Processes in the Development and Maintenance of Chronic Pain," *The Journal of Pain* 17, 9 Supplement (September 2016): T70–92.

31 Tatjana Barskova and Rainer Oesterreich, "Post-Traumatic Growth in People Living with a Serious Medical Condition and Its Relations to Physical and Mental Health: A Systematic Review," *Disability and Rehabilitation* 31, no. 21 (2009): 1709–33.

32 Carol S. Dweck, *Mindset: The New Psychology of Success* (New York: Random House, 2006).

33 Daniel C. Cherkin et al., "Effect of Mindfulness-Based Stress Reduction vs Cognitive Behavioral Therapy or Usual Care on Back Pain and Functional Limitations in Adults With Chronic Low Back Pain: A Randomized Clinical Trial," *The Journal of the American Medical Association* 315, no. 12 (March 22–29, 2016): 1240–49.

34 Elizabeth Andersen et al., "Effects of Mindfulness-Based Stress Reduction on Experimental Pain Sensitivity and Cortisol Responses in Women with Early Life Abuse: A Randomized Controlled Trial," *Psychosomatic Medicine* 83, no. 6 (July–August 2021): 515–27.

35 Maddalena Boccia, Laura Piccardi, and Paola Guariglia, "The Meditative Mind: A Comprehensive Meta-Analysis of MRI Studies," *Biomed Research International* 2015 (2015): 419808.

36 Fadal Zeidan, Jennifer N. Baumgartner, and Robert C. Coghill, "The Neural Mechanisms of Mindfulness-Based Pain Relief: A Functional Magnetic Resonance Imaging-Based Review and Primer," *Pain Reports* 4, no. 4 (August 7, 2019): e759.

37 Jared R. Lindahl, Nathan E. Fisher, David J. Cooper, Rochelle K. Rosen, Willoughby B. Britton, "The Varieties of Contemplative Experience: A Mixed-Methods Study of Meditation-Related Challenges in Western Buddhists," *PLoS One* (May 24, 2017).

38 I. Pilowsky, I. Crettenden, and M. Townley, "Sleep Disturbance in Pain Clinic Patients," *Pain* 23, no. 1 (September 1985): 27–33.

39 Jane L. Mathias, Megan L. Cant, and Anne L.J. Burke, "Sleep Disturbances and Sleep Disorders in Adults Living with Chronic Pain: A Meta-Analysis," *Sleep Medicine* 25 (December 2018): 198–210.

40 Adam J. Krause et al., "The Pain of Sleep Loss: A Brain Characterization in Humans," *The Journal of Neuroscience* 39, no. 12 (March 20, 2019): 2291–300.

41 Luciana Besedovsky, Tanja Lange, and Monika Haack, "The Sleep-Immune Crosstalk in Health and Disease," *Physiological Reviews* 99, no. 3 (July 1, 2019): 1325–80.

42 Ivy C. Mason et al., "Light Exposure During Sleep Impairs Cardiometabolic Function," *The Proceedings of the National Academy of Sciences* 119, no. 12 (March 22, 2022): e2113290119.

43 Alinny R. Isaac, Ricardo A.S. Lima-Filho, and Mychael V. Lourenco, "How Does the Skeletal Muscle Communicate with the Brain in Health and Disease?" *Neuropharmacology* 197, no. 1 (October 2021): 108744.

44 Katherinne Ferro Moura Franco et al., "Prescription of Exercises for the Treatment of Chronic Pain Along the Continuum of Nociplastic Pain: A Systematic Review with Meta-Analysis," *European Journal of Pain* 25, no. 1 (January 2021): 51–70; Louise J. Geneen et al., "Physical Activity and Exercise for Chronic Pain in Adults: An Overview of Cochrane Reviews," *Cochrane Database of Systematic Reviews* 4, no. 4 (April 24, 2017): CD011279; Patrick J. Owen et al., "Which Specific Modes of Exercise Training Are Most Effective for Treating Low Back Pain? Network Meta-Analysis," *British Journal of Sports Medicine* 54, no. 21 (November 2020): 1279–87; M. Dolores Sosa-Reina et al., "Effectiveness of Therapeutic Exercise in Fibromyalgia Syndrome: A Systematic Review and Meta-Analysis of Randomized Clinical

Trials," *Biomed Research International* 2017 (2017): 2356346; Feilong Zhu et al., "Yoga Compared to Non-Exercise or Physical Therapy Exercise on Pain, Disability, and Quality of Life for Patients with Chronic Low Back Pain: A Systematic Review and Meta-Analysis of Randomized Controlled Trials," *PLoS One* 15, no. 9 (September 1, 2020): e0238544.

45 Daniel L. Belavy et al., "Pain Sensitivity Is Reduced by Exercise Training: Evidence From a Systematic Review and Meta-Analysis," *Neuroscience & Biobehavioral Reviews* 120 (January 2021): 100–8.

46 Michael A. Wewege and Matthew D. Jones, "Exercise-Induced Hypoalgesia in Healthy Individuals and People with Chronic Musculoskeletal Pain: A Systematic Review and Meta-Analysis," *The Journal of Pain* 22, no. 1 (January 2021): 21–31.

47 Katherinne Ferro Moura Franco et al., "Prescription of Exercises for the Treatment of Chronic Pain Along the Continuum of Nociplastic Pain: A Systematic Review with Meta-Analysis," *European Journal of Pain* 25, no. 1 (January 2021): 51–70.

48 Özgül Öztürk et al., "Changes in Prefrontal Cortex Activation with Exercise in Knee Osteoarthritis Patients with Chronic Pain: An fNIRS Study," *Journal of Clinical Neuroscience* 90 (August 2021): 144–51.

49 Feilong Zhu et al., "Yoga Compared to Non-Exercise or Physical Therapy Exercise on Pain, Disability, and Quality of Life for Patients with Chronic Low Back Pain: A Systematic Review and Meta-Analysis of Randomized Controlled Trials," *PLoS One* 15, no. 9 (September 1, 2020): e0238544.

50 Carla Vanti et al., "The Effectiveness of Walking versus Exercise on Pain and Function in Chronic Low Back Pain: A Systematic Review and Meta-Analysis of Randomized Trials," *Disability and Rehabilitation* 41, no. 6 (March 2019): 622–32.

51 Kylie Isenburg et al., "Increased Salience Network Connectivity Following Manual Therapy Is Associated with Reduced Pain in Chronic Low Back Pain Patients," *The Journal of Pain* 22, no. 5 (May 2021): 545–55.

52 Julianne Holt-Lunstad, Timothy B. Smith, and J. Bradley Layton, "Social Relationships and Mortality Risk: A Meta-Analytic Review," *PLoS Medicine* 7, no. 7 (July 27, 2010): e1000316.

53 Helen P. Hailes et al., "Long-Term Outcomes of Childhood Sexual Abuse: An Umbrella Review," *The Lancet Psychiatry* 6, no. 10 (October 2019): 830–39; Etienne G. Krug et al., "The World Report on Violence and Health," *The Lancet* 360, no. 9339 (October 5, 2002): 1083–88; Ingrid Walker-Descartes et al., "Domestic Violence and Its Effects on Women, Children, and Families," *Pediatric Clinics of North America* 68, no. 2 (April 2021): 455–64.

54 James H. Fowler and Nicholas A. Christakis, "Dynamic Spread of Happiness in

a Large Social Network: Longitudinal Analysis Over 20 Years in the Framingham Heart Study," *The British Medical Journal* 337 (2008): a2338.

55 Mark P. Jensen et al., "Psychosocial Factors and Adjustment to Chronic Pain in Persons with Physical Disabilities: A Systematic Review," *Archives of Physical Medicine and Rehabilitation* 92, no. 1 (January 2011): 146–60.

56 Jean-Yves Rotge et al., "A Meta-Analysis of the Anterior Cingulate Contribution to Social Pain," *Social Cognitive and Affective Neuroscience* 10, no. 1 (January 2015): 19–27.

57 Gesa Berretz et al. "The Brain Under Stress: A Systematic Review and Activation Likelihood Estimation Meta-Analysis of Changes in BOLD Signal Associated with Acute Stress Exposure," *Neuroscience & Biobehavioral Reviews* 124 (May 2021): 89–99; Huiying Wang, Christoph Braun, and Paul Enck, "How the Brain Reacts to Social Stress (Exclusion): A Scoping Review," *Neuroscience & Biobehavioral Reviews* 80 (September 2017): 80–88.

58 Victoria D. Powell et al., "Bad Company: Loneliness Longitudinally Predicts the Symptom Cluster of Pain, Fatigue, and Depression in Older Adults," *Journal of the American Geriatrics Society* 70, no. 8 (August 2022): 2225–34.

59 Katerina V.-A. Johnson and Robin I.M. Dunbar, "Pain Tolerance Predicts Human Social Network Size," *Scientific Reports* 6 (2016): 25267.

60 Larissa L. Meijer et al., "Neural Basis of Affective Touch and Pain: A Novel Model Suggests Possible Targets for Pain Amelioration," *Journal of Neuropsychology* 16, no. 1 (March 2022): 38–53.

61 Jennifer Pierce et al., "Characterizing Pain and Generalized Sensory Sensitivity According to Trauma History Among Patients with Knee Osteoarthritis," *Annals of Behavioral Medicine* 55, no. 9 (August 23, 2021): 853–69.

62 C. Nathan Dewall et al. "Acetaminophen Reduces Social Pain: Behavioral and Neural Evidence," *Association for Psychological Science* 21, no. 7 (July 2010): 931–37.

63 Ben Carey et al., "Outcomes of a Controlled Trial with Visiting Therapy Dog Teams on Pain in Adults in an Emergency Department," *PLoS One* 17, no. 3 (March 9, 2022): e0262599.

64 Lois M. Verbrugge and Alan M. Jette, "The Disablement Process," *Social Science & Medicine* 38, no. 1 (1994): 1–14.

65 Patricia P. Katz and Edward H. Yelin, "Activity Loss and the Onset of Depressive Symptoms: Do Some Activities Matter More Than Others?" *Arthritis & Rheumatism* 44, no. 5 (May 2001): 1194–202.

66 Pim Cuijpers, Annemieke van Straten, and Lisanne Warmerdam, "Behavioral Activation Treatments of Depression: A Meta-Analysis," *Clinical Psychology Review* 27, no. 3 (April 2007): 318–26.

67 Klaus Munkholm, Asger Sand Paludan-Müller, and Kim Boesen, "Considering the Methodological Limitations in the Evidence Base of Antidepressants for Depression: A Reanalysis of a Network Meta-Analysis," *BMJ Open* 9, no. 6 (June 27, 2019): e024886; Andrea Cipriani et al., "Comparative Efficacy and Acceptability of 21 Antidepressant Drugs for the Acute Treatment of Adults with Major Depressive Disorder: A Systematic Review and Network Meta-Analysis," *The Lancet* 391, no. 10128 (April 7, 2018): 1357–66.

68 Barbara L. Fredrickson and Thomas Joiner, "Positive Emotions Trigger Upward Spirals Toward Emotional Well-Being," *Psychological Science* 13, no. 2 (March 2002): 172–25.

69 Mihaly Csikszentmihalyi, *Flow: The Psychology of Optimal Experience* (New York: Harper & Row, 1990). His name is pronounced something close to: me-HIGH chick-SENT-me-high-lee.

70 Susie Cranston and Scott Keller, "Increasing the 'Meaning Quotient' of Work," *McKinsey Quarterly* 1 (2013):48–59.

71 A. Ribaud et al., "Which Physical Activities and Sports Can Be Recommended to Chronic Low Back Pain Patients After Rehabilitation?" *Annals of Physical and Rehabilitation Medicine* 56, no. 7–8 (October 2013): 576–94.

72 www.uswitch.com/mobiles/screentime-report.

73 www.visiondirect.co.uk/blog/research-reveals-screen-time-habits.

74 Katherine Dahlsgaard, ChristopherPeterson, and Martin E.P. Seligman, "Shared Virtue: The Convergence of Valued Human Strengths Across Culture and History," *Review of General Psychology* 9, no. 3 (2005): 203–13.

75 Christopher Peterson and Martin E.P. Seligman, *Character Strengths and Virtues: A Handbook and Classification* (American Psychological Association; Oxford University Press, 2004).

76 Marianna Graziosi et al., "A Strengths-Based Approach to Chronic Pain," *The Journal of Positive Psychology* 17, no. 3 (2022): 400–8.

77 Angela L. Duckworth et al., "Grit: Perseverance and Passion for Long-Term Goals," *Journal of Personality and Social Psychology* 92, no. 6 (June 2007): 1087–101.

78 Tsubasa Kawasaki and Ryosuke Tozawa, "Grit in Community-Dwelling Older Adults with Low Back Pain Is Related to Self-Physical Training Habits," *Physical Medicine and Rehabilitation* 12, no. 10 (October 2020): 984–89.

79 Anna L. Boggiss et al., "A Systematic Review of Gratitude Interventions: Effects on Physical Health and Health Behaviors," *Journal of Psychosomatic Research* 135 (August 2020): 110165.

80 Marta Jackowska et al., "The Impact of a Brief Gratitude Intervention on Subjec-

tive Well-Being, Biology and Sleep," *Journal of Health Psychology* 21, no. 10 (October 2016): 2207–17.

81 Mary Janevic et al., "A Community Health Worker-Led Positive Psychology Intervention for African American Older Adults with Chronic Pain," *The Gerontologist* 62, no. 9 (November 2022): 1369–80.

82 Lee Rowland and Oliver Scott Curry, "A Range of Kindness Activities Boost Happiness," *The Journal of Social Psychology* 159, no. 3 (2019): 340–43.

83 Marc A. Musick, "Survey of Texas Adults, 2004" Inter-university Consortium for Political and Social Research (2005); Jerf W.K. Yeung, Zhuoni Zhang, and Tae Yeun Kim. "Volunteering and Health Benefits in General Adults: Cumulative Effects and Forms," *BMC Public Health* 18, article 8 (2018); published correction appears in *BMC Public Health* 17, article 736 (2017).

84 Elizabeth Salt, Leslie J. Crofford, and Suzanne Segerstrom, "The Mediating and Moderating Effect of Volunteering on Pain and Depression, Life Purpose, Well-Being, and Physical Activity," *Pain Management Nursing* 18, no. 4 (August 2017): 243–49.

85 Wendy J. Phillips and Donald W. Hine, "Self-Compassion, Physical Health, and Health Behaviour: A Meta-Analysis," *Health Psychology Review* 15, no. 1 (2021):113–39.

86 Xianglong Zeng et al., "The Effect of Loving-Kindness Meditation on Positive Emotions: A Meta-Analytic Review," *Frontiers in Psychology* 6 (November 3, 2015): 1693; Khoa D. Le Nguyen et al., "Loving-Kindness Meditation Slows Biological Aging in Novices: Evidence from a 12-Week Randomized Controlled Trial," *Psychoneuroendocrinology* 108 (October 2019): 20–27.

87 Summer Allen, "The Science of Awe," (white paper, Greater Good Science Center at UC Berkeley for the John Templeton Foundation, September 2018).

88 Ryota Takano and Michio Nomura, "Neural Representations of Awe: Distinguishing Common and Distinct Neural Mechanisms," *Emotion* 22, no. 4 (June 2022):669–77.

89 Matthew T. Ballew and Allen M. Omoto, "Absorption: How Nature Experiences Promote Awe and Other Positive Emotions," *Ecopsychology* 10, no. 1 (March 2018): 26–35.

90 Margaret M. Hansen, Reo Jones, and Kirsten Tocchini, "Shinrin-Yoku (Forest Bathing) and Nature Therapy: A State-of-the-Art Review," *International Journal of Environmental Research and Public Health* 14, no. 8 (August 2017): 851.

91 Qing Li et al., "Forest Bathing Enhances Human Natural Killer Activity and Expression of Anti-Cancer Proteins," *International Journal of Immunopathology and Pharmacology* 20, Supplement 2 (April–June 2007): 3–8.

92 Xindi Zhang, Yixin Zhang, and Jun Zhai, "Home Garden with Eco-Healing Functions Benefiting Mental Health and Biodiversity During and After the COVID-19 Pandemic: A Scoping Review," *Frontiers in Public Health* 9 (2021): 740187.

93 Celia Moreno-Morales et al., "Music Therapy in the Treatment of Dementia: A Systematic Review and Meta-Analysis," *Frontiers in Medicine* 7 (May 19, 2020): 160.

94 Jenny Hole et al., "Music as an Aid for Postoperative Recovery in Adults: A Systematic Review and Meta-Analysis," *The Lancet* 386, no. 10004 (October 24, 2015):1659–71; Tríona McCaffrey et al., "The Role and Outcomes of Music Listening for Women in Childbirth: An Integrative Review," *Midwifery* 83 (April 2020): 102627; Eduardo A. Garza-Villarreal et al., "Music-Induced Analgesia in Chronic Pain Conditions: A Systematic Review and Meta-Analysis," *Pain Physician* 20, no. 7 (November 2017): 597–610.

95 Töres Theorell, "Links Between Arts and Health, Examples from Quantitative Intervention Evaluations," *Frontiers in Psychology* 12 (December 14, 2021): 12:742032.

96 Carolyn E. Schwartz CE et al., "Doing Good, Feeling Good, and Having More: Resources Mediate the Health Benefits of Altruism Differently for Males and Females with Lumbar Spine Disorders," *Applied Research in Quality of Life* 7, no. 3 (2012): 263–79.

97 Pew Research Center, "The Global Religious Landscape: A Report on the Size and Distribution of the World's Major Religious Groups as of 2010," The Pew Forum on Religion & Public Life (December 2012).

98 Tyler J. VanderWeele, Tracy A. Balboni, Howard H. Koh, "Health and Spirituality," *The Journal of the American Medical Association* 318, no. 6 (August 8, 2017): 519–20.

99 Alexandra Ferreira-Valente et al., "The Role of Spirituality in Pain, Function, and Coping in Individuals with Chronic Pain," *Pain Medicine* 21, no. 3 (March 1, 2020): 448–57.

100 Eric S. Kim et al., "Sense of Purpose in Life and Likelihood of Future Illicit Drug Use or Prescription Medication Misuse," *Psychosomatic Medicine* 82, no. 7 (September 2020): 715–21.

101 Brandon L. Boring et al., "Meaning in Life and Pain: The Differential Effects of Coherence, Purpose, and Mattering on Pain Severity, Frequency, and the Development of Chronic Pain," *Journal of Pain Research* 15 (February 3, 2022): 299–314.

102 Randy Cohen, Chirag Bavishi, and Alan Rozanski, "Purpose in Life and Its Relationship to All-Cause Mortality and Cardiovascular Events: A Meta-Analysis," *Psychosomatic Medicine* 78, no. 2 (February–March 2016): 122–33.

103 Kevin W. Chen et al., A Pilot Study of External Qigong Therapy for Patients with Fibromyalgia," *The Journal of Alternative and Complementary Medicine* 12, no. 9 (November 2006): 851–56.

104 Eleanor Ratcliffe, Birgitta Gatersleben, and Paul T. Sowden, "Associations with Bird Sounds: How Do They Relate to Perceived Restorative Potential?" *Journal of Environmental Psychology* 47 (2016): 136–44.

105 Yoni K. Ashar et al., "Effect of Pain Reprocessing Therapy vs Placebo and Usual Care for Patients with Chronic Back Pain: A Randomized Clinical Trial," *JAMA Psychiatry* 79, no. 1 (2022): 13–23.

106 Marsha M. Linehan, *DBT Skills Training Handouts and Worksheets,* 2nd edition (New York: Guilford Press, 2015).

107 Everett L. Worthington, *Five Steps to Forgiveness: The Art and Science of Forgiving* (New York: Crown, 2001).

RESOURCES

Professional Help

American College of Rheumatology (patients and caregivers)
rheumatology.org/I-Am-A/Patient-Caregiver

American Psychological Association
locator.apa.org
To find a therapist, enter your city and state and plug in "pain management."

Arthritis Foundation
Arthritis.org

Domestic Violence Hotline
(800) 799-7233, (800) 787-3224 (TTY), or TheHotline.org

National Academy of Medicine Chronic Pain Journey Map
nam.edu/programs/action-collaborative-on-countering-the-u-s-opioid-epidemic/
  chronic-pain-journey-map

National Human Trafficking Resource Center
(888) 373-7888 (TTY: 711)

Substance Abuse Helpline
(800) 662-HELP (4357)

Suicide & Crisis Lifeline
988 or 988lifeline.org

US Pain Foundation
USPainFoundation.org

Pain Self-Management

AftonHassett.com
Click on the Resources tab for videos and recordings for guided imagery, meditations, progressive muscle relaxation, and breathing techniques. You'll also find the *Chronic Pain Reset* podcast on my website.

Happify.com
Excellent evidenced-based resources here can help improve well-being and life satisfaction in chronic illness.

PainGuide.com
On this open-access website, you can find a remarkable array of information and support for learning more about chronic pain and the skills and practices you need to thrive.

ThePainTools.com
Guided and personalized pain self-care delivered in an innovative way.

Books

Dahl, JoAnne, and Tobias Lundgren. *Living Beyond Your Pain: Using Acceptance and Commitment Therapy to Ease Chronic Pain.* Oakland, CA: New Harbinger, 2006.

Gordon, Alan, and Alon Ziv. *The Way Out: A Revolutionary, Scientifically Proven Approach to Healing Chronic Pain.* New York: Avery, 2021.

Hayes, Steven C., and Spencer Smith. *Get Out of Your Mind and Into Your Life: The New Acceptance and Commitment Therapy.* Oakland, CA: New Harbinger, 2005.

Kabot-Zinn, Jon. *The Healing Power of Mindfulness: A New Way of Being.* New York: Hachette Books, 2018.

Kross, Ethan. *Chatter: The Voice in Our Head, Why It Matters, and How to Harness It.* New York: Crown, 2021.

Linehan, Marsha M. *DBT Skills Training Handouts and Worksheets,* 2nd edition. New York: Guilford Press, 2015.

McEwen, Bruce, and Elizabeth Norton Lasley. (2002). *The End of Stress as We Know It.* Washington, DC: Joseph Henry Press, 2002.

Neff, Kristin. *Self-Compassion: The Proven Power of Being Kind to Yourself.* New York: William Morrow, 2011.

Sapolsky, Robert M. *Why Zebras Don't Get Ulcers: A Guide to Stress, Stress-Related Diseases, and Coping.* New York: W.H. Freeman, 1994.

Schubiner, Howard, and Michael Betzold. *Unlearn Your Pain: A 28-Day Process to Reprogram Your Brain,* 4th edition. Pleasant Ridge, MI: Mind Body Publishing, 2022.

Strecher, Victor J. *Life on Purpose: How Living for What Matters Most Changes Everything.* New York: HarperOne, 2016.

van der Kolk, Bessel. *The Body Keeps the Score: Brain, Mind, and Body in the Healing of Trauma.* New York: Viking, 2014.

Weaver, Stephanie. *The Migraine Relief Plan Cookbook: More Than 100 Anti-Inflammatory Recipes for Managing Headaches and Living a Healthier Life.* Evanston, IL: Agate Surrey, 2022.

Wood, Wendy. *Good Habits, Bad Habits: The Science of Making Positive Changes That Stick.* New York: Farrar, Straus and Giroux, 2019.

INDEX

A

abusive relationships, 88
acceptance and commitment therapy
    (ACT), 176–77
acetaminophen, 91–92
activity pacing, 82, 101–2, 164–65
activity trackers, 233
adrenaline, 71
adversity. *See also* trauma
    making sense of, 56–57
    personal failures, 55–56
    professional help for, 53, 54
    serious types of, 53
Ahrens, Ben, 12–13
Allen, Summer, 126
allostatic load, 29
altruism, 131
amygdala, 24, 42
amygdala hijack, 43
Andwele, Michele, 149–50
antibodies, 26
antidepressants, 100
anxiety
    associated with chronic pain conditions,
        16

compared with depression, 65
    and negative thoughts, 36
    neural circuitry studies, 42
arts, and healing effects, 129–31, 204–5
autonomic nervous system, 25
awe, power of, 126–33, 210–11

B

bacterial infections, 16–17, 26
Ballew, Matthew, 128
blood pressure, 28
Boccia, Maddalena, 65
body scan, 63
Boehnke, Kevin, 58–59
bone loss, 79
Boring, Brandon, 138, 139
bottom-up pain, 8–10, 77
brain. *See also* top-down pain
    emotion-processing areas, 34
    how it processes awe, 127
    how it processes pain, 4–5
    impact of thoughts on, 34–40
    and mindfulness practices, 65
    neural circuitry, 42

brain (*continued*)
  plasticity, 7–8
  reward processing system, 47–48,
    127
  sensitized, symptoms of, 6–7
Brandl, Felix, 42
breathing
  mindful, 156–57
  in mindfulness practices, 63
  paced, 152–53
broaden and build theory of positive
    emotions, 46

C
cancer pain, xvii
Carey, Ben, 92
catastrophic thoughts, 38–39, 54
central nervous system, 25
character strengths, 106–15
*Character Strengths and Virtues: A Hand-
    book and Classification*, 107
character survey, 115
Chatter (Kross), 37
Chen, Kevin, 142
Cherkin, Daniel, 64
Christakis, Nicholas, 88
chronic inflammation, 26–27
chronic low back pain
  brain-generated, 43–45
  depression and anxiety from, 16
  exercising with, 101
  experienced by John F. Kennedy, 19
  MBSR therapy for, 64
  research studies on, 217
  yoga for, 79

chronic pain. *See also* chronic low back
    pain; fibromyalgia; pain manage-
    ment strategies
  antiquated ideas about, 5–6, 15–19
  catastrophic thoughts about, 38–39
  common chronic conditions, 14
  co-occurring conditions and symp-
    toms, 14–21
  good and bad days, 97–98, 236–37
  impact of loneliness, 89–90
  impact of negative emotions, 41–42
  impact of social exclusion, 88–90
  impact of toxic stress, 28–29
  leading to pain avoidance, 39
  leading to social withdrawal, 91–92
  link with depression, 84
  link with sleep disturbances, 69
  medical interventions for, 216–17
  SPACE symptoms, 19–21
  symptom trackers, 233–34
  talking about, 193
  unique neural signature, 42
  and weakened reward-processing
    system, 47–48
Chronic Pain and Fatigue Research Cen-
    ter (CPFRC), 5–6
circadian rhythms, 72
Clauw, Dan, 5, 14–15, 58
cognitive behavioral therapy (CBT)
  emotion-focused, 45
  goal of, 174
  next-generation therapies, 39, 43
  scientific evidence for, 34–36
  temporal order and causality in, 34
cognitive errors, 37
coherence, idea of, 138

community, criteria for, 90

complex regional pain syndrome (CRPS), 104–5

connection, daily, 192–93

cortisol, 28

courage, 109–10

Cranston, Susie, 101

Csikszentmihalyi, Mihaly, 100–101

Curry, Oliver Scott, 120

Cyberball, 89

cytokines, 17, 27

D

daily social connection, 192–93

dance therapy, 79–80

dentistry, 18

deployment, 39–40

depression
  compared with anxiety, 65
  easing, with pleasant activities, 99–100
  link with chronic pain, 16, 84
  link with negative thoughts, 36
  from loss of VLAs, 98–99
  neural circuitry studies, 42
  professional help for, xvii, 136

Deuble, John, 84–85

Dewall, Nathan, 91

dialectical behavior therapy (DBT), 182–83, 184

diaries and journals
  device diary, 102
  gratitude journal, 201
  sleep diary, 72–73

disabled people, 95

dogs, 92–93

domains
  in daily activities section, 147–48
  in Thriving Plan, 219

dopamine, 47

drug use, 137

Duckworth, Angela, 117

Dweck, Carol, 56, 118

E

eating, mindful, 63–64

electronic devices, 102–3

emotional awareness and expression therapy (EAET), 45

emotional flooding reaction, 43

emotion-processing areas, 34

emotions, negative
  arising from tortured thoughts, 71
  biological consequences of, 41–42
  emotion-focused therapies for, 45
  mindfulness therapy for, 63
  releasing, 184–85
  survival value of, 46

emotions, positive
  benefits of, 46–47
  broaden and build theory of, 46
  embracing, 186–87
  evasiveness of, 41–42
  inability to recognize, 47–48
  upward spiral created by, 100

endocrine system, 47

endorphins, 47, 76

The End of Stress as We Know It (McEwen), 27

exercise, 76–83
  activity pacing, 82, 101–2, 164–65

exercise (*continued*)
　　aerobic, 78–79
　　brain changes from, 78
　　choosing type of, 78
　　for chronic low back pain, 101
　　dance therapy, 79–80
　　for easing pain sensitivity, 77–78
　　finding time for, 82–83
　　for flexibility, 79
　　on good and bad days, 81–82
　　high- and low-impact, 78
　　mind-body, benefits of, 79
　　overdoing it, 81–82
　　physical benefits, 76–77
　　physical therapy (PT), 80–81
　　psychological benefits, 77
　　self-directed, 117–18
　　setting goals for, 81
　　strength training, 79
　　stretching exercises, 63
　　time-based activity pacing, 82
　　walking, 80
expectations, managing, 139

F
failures, 55–56
fibromyalgia
　　depression and anxiety from, 16
　　diagnosing, 18
　　pain sensitivity with, 7
　　research on, 14
　　sleep patterns with, 71
　　symptoms of, 58–59
FIERCE, 89
fight-flight-or-freeze response, 6, 24,
　　25–26, 42–43

fixed mindset, 56
*Flow: The Psychology of Optimal
　　Experience* (Csikszentmihalyi),
　　100–101
forest bathing, 128
forgiveness, 194–95
Fowler, James, 88
Framingham Heart Study, 88
Fredrickson, Barbara, 46, 100
Full Catastrophe Living (Kabat-Zinn),
　　156

G
Gay, Monica, 124–25
generalized sensory sensitivity, 6, 91
giving, the gift of, 198–99
Goleman, Daniel, 43
golf, 80, 101–2
Good Habits, Bad Habits (Wood), 234
grace, 120–23
gratitude, 118–19, 200–201
gratitude journal, 201
Graziosi, Marianna, 113
grief, 56–57
grit, 116–18
growth mindset, 56, 118
grudges, 194–95
guided imagery, 67, 158–59

H
habits, establishing, 234–35
Habit Stacking (Scott), 234
Hale, Elizabeth, 20
happiness clustering, 88
happiness messengers, 47

Harte, Steve, 5, 19

Hayes, Steven, 176

HEAL initiative Back Pain Consortium
(HEAL BACPAC), 217

Heartfelt Compliment, 193

highly sensitive persons (HSP), 6–7

hobbies, 67

Holt-Lunstad, Julianne, 86

horticultural therapy, 129

humanity, 109

human touch, 90

hypothalamus, 24

I

Identify, Connect, Feel, Accept, Reset
(ICFAR), 185

immune system

reaction to fight-flight-or-freeze, 26

response to infections, 17

strengthening, with forest bathing,
128–29

strengthening, with self-compassion,
122

weakened, from poor sleep, 70

imperfections, embracing, 55, 225

infections, 16–17, 26

inflammation, 26–27

Insight Timer, 67

insomnia

acute, statistics on, 69

causes of, 70–71

effect on immune system, 70

effect on pain sensitivity, 70

link with chronic pain, 69

interoception, 6

Isenburg, Kylie, 81

J

Jackowska, Marta, 119

James, William, 45

Janevic, Mary, 119

Jensen, Mark, 88

justice, 110–11

K

Kabat-Zinn, Jon, 61, 156

Kaplan, Chelsea, 16

Kattari, Shanna Katz, 95–96

Katz, Patricia, 98

Keller, Scott, 101

Kennedy, John F., 19

Kim, Eric, 137

kindness, 120–23, 196–97

Krause, Adam, 70

Kross, Ethan, 37

L

Lehrer, Paul, 152

Life on Purpose (Strecher), 207

lifestyle activity exercise, 82–83

light exposure, 72

Lindahl, Jarad, 66

Lived Experiences

Ben Ahrens, 12–13

Cassandra Metzger, 31–32

Christin Veasley, 49–50

Cynthia Toussaint, 104–5

John Deuble, 84–85

Kathleen Sutherland, 134–35

Kevin Boehnke, 58–59

Lynne Kennedy Matallana, 224–25

Michele Andwele, 149–50

Lived Experiences (*continued*)
  Monica Gay, 124–25
  Shanna Katz Kattari, 95–96
loneliness, 89–90
loving-kindness meditation, 122
lupus, 95
Lyme disease, 12–13

M
manual physical therapy, 81
Matallana, Lynne Kennedy, 224–25
mattering, concept of, 138
McEwen, Bruce, 27, 87
McKernan, Lindsey, 235–36
McMillan, David, 90
medial temporal lobes, 42
medications, 10, 84
meditation
  history of, 66
  loving-kindness, 122
  mindfulness, 63
  negative effects associated with, 66
  pain relief from, 31–32
  walking, 63
mental health providers, xvii, 53, 54, 136
mental time travel, 64–65
meta-analysis, 48
Metzger, Cassandra, 31–32
Military Academy at West Point, 117
mindful breathing, 156–57
mindful eating, 63–64
mindfulness-based stress reduction
  (MBSR), 60–67
mindfulness meditation, 63
mindful walking, 66–67
Miserandino, Christine, 95

mixed-pain condition, 10
monkey mind, 61
multifactorial genetic inheritance disorders, 23
muscle relaxation, progressive, 154–55
music, 129–30, 188–89
myokines, 77

N
naps, 73
natural killer cells, 128–29
nature and awe, 127–29
nature breaks, 170–71
Neff, Kristin, 172
negative thoughts
  emotion-focused therapies for, 45
  mindfulness therapy for, 63
  reframing, 174–75
  repercussions of, 36–39
  unhelpful, 36–39, 63
negativity bias, 40
nervous system, 25
neural circuitry, 42
neuroplasticity, xv
Newbold, Dillan, 8
Niemiec, Ryan, 113
nociplastic pain, 8, 9. *See also* top-down
  pain
Nomura, Michio, 127

O
Omoto, Allen, 128
One More Question, 193
opioids, 84
optimism, pragmatic, 39–40

orthopedics, 17–18

osteoarthritis, 78

oxytocin, 47, 92

P

paced breathing, 152–53

pain. *See also* chronic pain; pain management activities; pain management strategies; top-down pain

  bottom-up, 8–10, 77

  heightened sensitivity to, 6

  how brain processes, 4–5

  mixed-pain condition, 10

  "nociplastic," 8, 9

  physical, avoiding, 39

  understanding purposes of, 124–25

pain management activities

  about, 145–46

  acts of kindness, 196–97

  appreciating the arts, 204–5

  creating a relationship tree, 190–91

  cultivating purpose in life, 206–7

  embracing positive emotions, 186–87

  engaging in positive service, 202–3

  FAQs, 147–48

  forgiveness, 194–95

  the gift of giving, 198–99

  guided imagery, 158–59

  healthy sleep habits, 162–63

  imagining best possible self, 208–9

  listening to music, 188–89

  making daily connections, 192–93

  mindful breathing, 156–57

  paced breathing, 152–53

  pleasant activity scheduling, 166–67

  practicing gratitude, 200–201

  practicing self-compassion, 172–73

  progressive muscle relaxation, 154–55

  releasing painful emotions, 184–85

  savoring, 160–61

  self-soothing, 182–83

  taking a nature break, 170–71

  taking an "aweliday," 210–11

  thought approach 1: reframing negative thoughts, 174–75

  thought approach 2: unhelpful thoughts come and go, 176–77

  thought approach 3: coping coach, 178–79

  thought approach 4: somatic tracking, 180–81

  time-based pacing, 164–65

  walking program, 168–69

pain management strategies. *See also* pain management activities

  changing negative thought patterns, 35–39

  embracing failures and imperfections, 55–57

  embracing power of awe, 126–33

  emotion-focused CBT, 45

  exercise, 76–83

  having a strong sense of purpose, 137–41

  improving sleep quality, 73–75

  maintaining a growth mindset, 56

  mindfulness-based stress reduction (MBSR), 60–67

  positive emotions, 46–48

  practicing grit, gratitude, and grace, 116–23

  pragmatic optimism, 39–40

  prioritizing VALs, 98–103

pain management strategies (*continued*)
  qigong therapy, 142–44
  relying on values, virtues, and
    strengths, 106–15
  strengthening social ties, 87–94
pain reprocessing therapy (PRT),
    180–81
parasympathetic nervous system,
    24–25, 26
passion, 117
perfectionism, 224–25, 230
peripheral nervous system, 25
perseverance, 110, 113–14, 117
pets, 92–93
photography, 50
physical therapy (PT), 80–81
Pierce, Jennifer, 91
pleasant activity scheduling, 166–67
Positive Piggy Bank, 186–87
positive psychology, 107
positive service, 202–3
post-traumatic growth, 54–55
post-traumatic stress disorder (PTSD), 53
Powell, Victoria, 89
pragmatic optimism, 39–40
prayer, 125
prefrontal cortex, 78
prescription drugs, 137
present moment, existing in the, 61–62
progressive muscle relaxation, 154–55
psychiatric disorders, 14–21, 88, 107
purpose, cultivating, 206–7
purpose, power of, 137–41

Q
qigong therapy, 142–44

R
REACH model for forgiveness, 195
reappraisal, 65
relationship tree, 190–91
reminders, 232–33
resiliency, 53
restless leg syndrome, 69, 73
reward processing system, 47–48
rheumatoid arthritis, 98
rheumatology, 17
Rowland, Lee, 120
rumination, 65
Ryff, Carol, 137

S
Salt, Elizabeth, 121
savoring activity, 160–61
scars, embracing, 55
Schrepf, Andrew, 16, 19
Scott, Steve, 234
screen hours, 102–3
self-awareness, 65
self-compassion
  countering loss and despair with, 54
  effect on immune system, 122
  quieting your inner critic with, 38, 236
  in Thriving Plan, 172–73
  what it means, 121–22
self-denial, 149–50
self-directed exercise, 117–18
selflessness, 131
self-regulation, 65
self-soothe activity, 182–83
sensory sensitivity, generalized, 6, 91
serotonin, 47
Shaikh, Sana, 22–23

shinrin yoku, 128

sickness cytokines, 17, 27

Sigal, Len, 142

sleep

    apnea, 69, 73

    healthy habits, 73–74, 162–63

    insomnia, 69–71

    naps, 73

    recording, in diary, 72–73

    -wake cycle, 72

sleep time stabilization, 75

social connectedness, 86–94

social encounters, painful, 35–36

social exclusion or rejection, 88–90,
    91–92

social media, 102

social sensitivity, 91

social withdrawal, 36, 91–92, 99

somatic nervous system, 25

somatic tracking, 180–81

SPACE profile, creating a, 21

SPACE symptoms, 19–21

spiritual development, 124–25

spirituality and awe, 131–32

Spoon Theory, 95–96

startle response, 42–43

Steptoe, Andrew, 119

Strecher, Vic, 137, 207

strength training, 79

stress

    chronic inflammation from, 26–27

    environmental triggers, 23–24

    good, normal, 27–28

    identifying sources of, 29

    stress-response system, 24–27, 71

    thinking about how you cope with,
        29–30

    from threats (startle response),
        42–43

    tolerable, 28

    toxic, 28–29, 60

    treating, with MBSR, 60–67

    triggered by by false alarms, 25–26,
        42–43

    vulnerability-stress model of human
        health, 23–24

stretching exercises, 63

support people, 235

survival, research on, 86

survival instinct, 93

Sutherland, Kathleen, 134–35

sympathetic nervous system, 24–25

symptom trackers, 233–34

T

Takano, Ryota, 127

temperance, 111–12

Text to Connect, 192–93

Theorell, Tores, 130

thought approach 1: reframing negative
    thoughts, 174–75

thought approach 2: unhelpful thoughts
    come and go, 176–77

thought approach 3: coping coach,
    178–79

thought approach 4: somatic tracking,
    180–81

thoughts. *See also* negative thoughts

    catastrophic, 38–39, 54

    coping, how they work, 178–79

    effect on brain, 34–40

    emotional, behavioral, and physiologi-
        cal reactions to, 34–36

thoughts (*continued*)
    emotions triggered by, 71
    power of, 33–34
    pragmatic optimism, 39–40
    unhelpful and automatic, 36–39,
        176–77
Thriving Plan. *See also* pain management
        activities
    blank worksheet, 223
    creating your own, 215–23
    guiding principles, 218
    key domains and activities, 219
    sample worksheet, 221
    working and living with, 230–37
time-based activity pacing, 82,
    164–65
tiny achievable goals (TAGs), 232
top-down pain
    about, 8–10
    best exercise for, 77
    common chronic conditions, 9
    example of, 43–45
    following infectious diseases,
        26–27
    multifactorial genetic inheritance
        disorders, 23
    overlapping symptoms, 16–19
Toussaint, Cynthia, 104–5
transcendence, 112–13
trauma
    effect on DNA, 42
    effect on social interactions, 91
    effect on world view, 54
    post-traumatic growth from,
        54–55
    professional help for, 53, 54
    rebounding from, 53
    research on, 53

U

US Army soldiers, 39–40
US Military, 116–17

V

vaccines, 70
valued life activities (VLAs), 98–100
values, virtues and strengths, 106–15
Vanti, Carla, 80
Veasley, Christin, 49–50
Verbrugge, Lois, 98
VIA (Values in Action) Institute on Char-
    acter, 107, 115
virtues values, and strengths, 106–15
viruses, 16–17, 26
visioning exercises, 208–9
visual arts, 130
volunteer work, 120–21, 202–3
vulnerability-stress model of human
    health, 23–24

W

wabi-sabi, 55
Waitley, Denis, 40
Walker, Matthew, 70
walking
    incorporating into your life, 80
    mindful, 66–67
    program, establishing a, 168–69
    walking meditation, 63
weight gain, 28
West Point Military Academy, 117
Williams, David, 5, 19, 235
wisdom, 108–9
Wood, Wendy, 234
Worthington, Everitt, 194–95

Y

Yellen, Ed, 98
yoga, 31–32, 59, 79
yogi breathing practices, 152

Z

Zee, Phyllis, 72
Zeidan, Fadel, 65
zest, 110, 113–14